Doctor Sebi Diet

The Complete Guide to Cleanse Liver, Blood and Intestine. Prevent Diseases with Approved Alkaline Food and Tasty Recipes for Detox, Weight Loss and Boost Your Health.

(2 Books in 1)

Lauren Hill

Table of Contents

Book 1

Doctor SEBI:

The Ultimate Diet to Cleanse Liver, Blood and Intestine with Alkaline Food, Herbs and Fasting. Detox your Body, Lose Weight and Restore your Energy.

Lauren Hill

INTRODUCTION

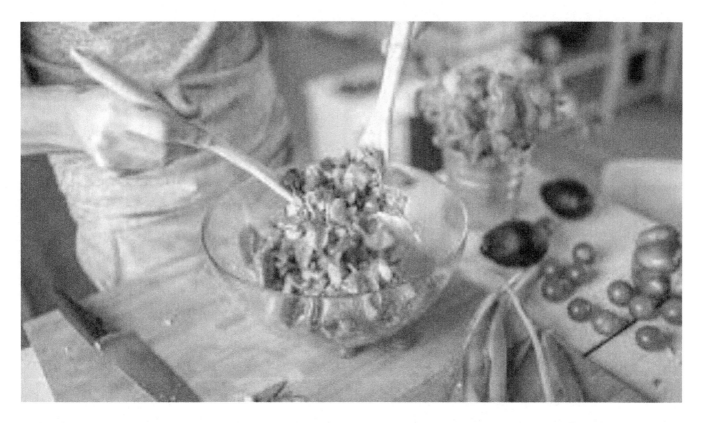

The Light and Love Journey (Dr. Sebi's Vision)

The alkaline diet is a revolutionary diet known as the alkaline ash diet or the acid-alkaline diet. This diet teaches that you can alter the amount of alkalinity or acidity in your body by merely adjusting the types of foods you eat.

Your metabolism is the process that turns the food you eat into energy for your body, and it is often compared to a fire in a furnace. Each of the processes involves a reaction between chemicals meant to break down a mass of solids. There is a kind of slow control to your body's chemical reactions, not like the raging inferno that a fire can become, but both processes leave a by-product known as ash. In the body, this ash is called metabolic waste, and it can be neutral, alkaline, or acidic, depending on the food you are consuming.

Who Is Dr. Sebi?

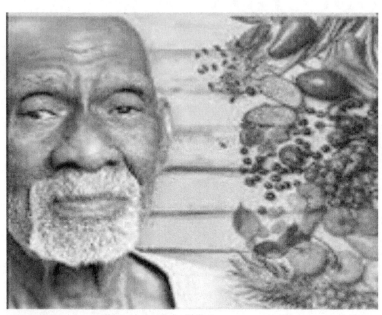

Dr. Sebi learned everything he needed to know about healing the human body through personal experience. He learned much about life by always studying the things he saw and heard and trying new ways to improve basic life. He was a naturalist who studied biochemistry, pathology, and herbs to create his unique health and wellness methodology. When traditional medical treatments did not heal his many ailments, he turned to the knowledge of a trained herbalist, looking for something to cure his obesity, asthma, and diabetes. He began experimenting with cell food compounds made from natural vegetation with the things he learned from the herbalist. His goal was to find foods that would cleanse the body on a cellular level. Inspired by his own healed body and the success he saw with his first few followers, Dr. Sebi began sharing his findings with others and called his creations 'Dr. Sebi's Cell Food'.

His methods focused on eating natural plant-based foods and herbs that are alkaline and avoiding hybrid acidic foods that can damage your body. He focused on teaching people to eat plant foods to minimize their bodies' acidity and prevent the buildup of compounds that cause disease and unhealthiness. The diet helps create an environment in the alkaline body to make it difficult for diseases to live.

What Is the Alkaline Diet?

Many of the familiar foods that you eat will cause your body to produce harmful acids. When you consume particular foods and beverages, they can change your body's acid levels and make your body more alkaline. Acid or alkaline is measured by comparing it to the levels on a pH scale, where the numbers measure readings from acid to alkaline, on a scale from zero to fourteen. The numbers from seven to fourteen are in the alkaline part of the scale.

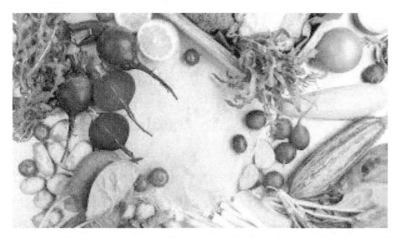

Changing your body's pH level from an acid to an alkaline can help you lose weight. If one of your body systems has an imbalance, it will let your brain know that something is wrong. The two systems that most often send messages to your mind are your stomach and urinary tract. Since they are used several times each day, they get a lot of workout from their food. When your stomach is not balanced, you might suffer from poor digestion, erratic mood swings, and low energy levels. It is essential to keep your stomach and intestines functioning at their peak performance since they do such a necessary job for you every day.

Your stomach is the first organ that your body uses to metabolize your body's food for energy. The stomach does this by secreting acids that help break down the food you eat while your abdomen churn to food to complete the process. If your stomach is not healthy, it will not digest your food correctly, and your entire body will be thrown off balance. The nutrition of the alkaline diet are designed to avoid the problems that come with system imbalances. When the food you eat is more alkaline, it will help neutralize the stomach acids to only digest your food and not the lining of your stomach. The main problem with acid in the stomach is that it doesn't come from just the stomach secretions and the food you eat, thus making the acid level more than the stomach can comfortably handle. When you avoid acidic foods and concentrate on alkaline foods, then you will allow your stomach to focus on healthy digestion as it begins to heal.

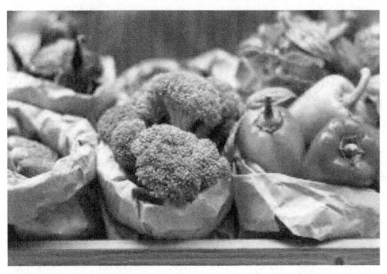

Scientific research shows that various foods will affect your body in multiple ways. The focus was specifically on the stomach and the kidneys, since everything you eat or drink will eventually pass through the stomach and then the kidneys. Certain foods are known to raise the pH levels of your body. The level of pH measures the number of hydrogen ions found in a specific amount of a substance. Your body needs hydrogen ions to keep the proteins in your body linked in the shape they need to stay in to fulfill their particular function. The proteins in your body have many essential functions. They carry nutrients to your cells as well as providing structure and support for your cells. They carry messages between the cells in the brain and the body. They assist the body in creating antibodies that will help fight off infection and disease. The hydrogen ions in your body will not perform the job they need to do if your body is too acidic, because then the hydrogen ions will not be strong enough to do their job. When your regular diet is rich in healthy alkaline foods will keep your body's pH level at a level that will support the work of the hydrogen ions.

Eating the recommended foods of the Alkaline Diet will promote a healthy environment inside of your body. It is almost an alternate form of medicine because the food choices you make will heal your body.

The Alkaline Diet offers smart food choices that will balance your body's pH level. When the pH level is correct in your body, your body will function properly the way it was meant to work.

How Does the Alkaline Diet Work?

Keeping the pH level of your body, and your blood, at an optimum level is essential so that your body will function properly. Your body works hard to keep the pH level of your blood around 7.4, which is at the beginning of the alkaline part of the scale. Your red blood cells float through your bloodstream and carry oxygen to your cells. The red blood cells have a protective coating that has an essential function in your body's health. As the cells move through your bloodstream, they will eventually come to tiny capillaries that need to have oxygen brought to them, but they are too small for the red blood cells to continue traveling in a group. At this point, the red blood cells must separate and stay apart, and the protective covering gives them the ability to do this by neutralizing their attractive charge. If the pH level in your blood is too acidic, it will destroy the protective coating on the red blood cells and make them stick together, so certain parts of your body will not be able to get supplies of oxygen-rich blood. And while the red blood cells are clumping together, they will eventually begin to die from lack of oxygen. Your body depends on an adequate supply of healthy red blood cells to be able to survive. And with less oxygen flowing to the cells of your body, your energy levels will plummet.

Every primary system in your body has its pH level to maintain. Keeping the pH levels of the body separate but functioning together is carefully maintained by your respiratory system, renal system, and your buffering system. The buffering system controls the proteins that are so important to the functioning of your body. This system also helps to keep all of the systems in your body balanced and running smoothly.

Your respiratory system regulates the intake of oxygen and the output of carbon dioxide. You take in oxygen and put out carbon dioxide with every breath that you take. Carbon dioxide is a waste product collected from your red blood cells, which they bring back after delivering the oxygen to your cells. Your renal system controls the pH level of the fluid around your cells and organs. Your body is continuously undergoing changes and adjustments to keep all of your pH levels in balance.

The Alkaline Diet helps you to keep all of your pH levels in balance. Your pH will affect every part of your body, especially if the levels are not in balance. Even after you have enjoyed a good night of sleep, you may awake to feel exhausted. Your gums and teeth might be sensitive, and they might even bleed. Your neck and shoulders will feel stiff and sore. You can suffer from frequent sinus symptoms, allergies, and from headaches for no real reason. Your joints will be stiff, not just in the morning, and they will hurt when made to bend or support you. You will probably experience shortness of breath even with gentle physical activity. Since your hormones will be too out of balance, you might experience acne, eczema, and yeast infections. Your skin will always feel dry. You will be irritable and depressed and suffer bouts of brain fog. Viruses seem to follow you around and just won't go away.

The Alkaline Diet is meant to help you correct all of these health issues. By filling your body full of right alkaline foods and avoiding the acidic foods that can wreck your health, you will not only lose weight and look better, but you will also feel better. The diet emphasizes regular healthy eating. You will eat more fruits, vegetables, whole grains, and you will stay well hydrated. You will cut back or eliminate meat, alcohol, sugar, and processed foods. Adherents of the Alkaline Diet know that consuming foods that cause acid in your body will lead to poor health because your pH levels are unbalanced. When you eat foods that make you healthy and keep you healthy, you will be healthy.

Chapter 1

HOLISTIC HEALING

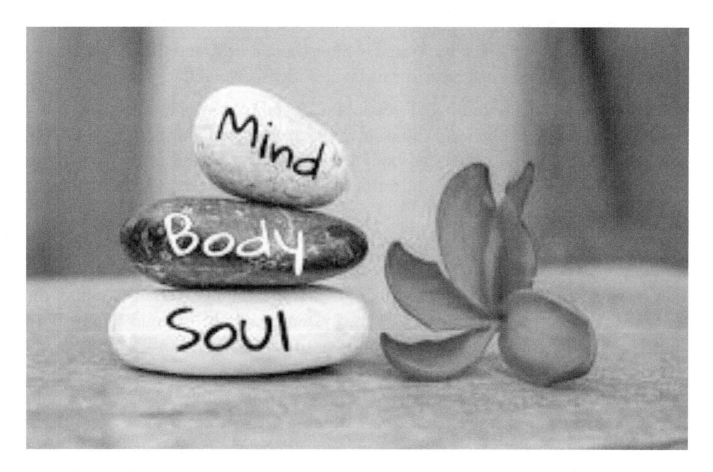

Mind, Body, and Spirit in Perfect Harmony

All of the essential ingredients can create powerful outcomes when focused inside the USA. However, when these elements are appropriately calibrated within the process for self-hypnosis, their effectiveness has magnified a hundredfold. Self-hypnosis is a process for creating your reality.

You might think that sounds magical or too great to be right, but that is relative to what you have gotten up for this point in your lifetime. These ideas could be relatively new to you.

Following is a fantastic example of the "relative" personality of new thoughts. Imagine that you are provided with a private jet that is beautifully outfitted with lavish appointments in addition to a well-trained crew. It is a beautiful gift, and you get to disclose this tech marvel to men and women not having ever seen anything like this.

Let us assume your pilot takes you back in time to before December 17, 1903, when the Wright Brothers announced their first flight in Kitty Hawk. You are pleased to show this miracle of technology to the Wright Brothers, who have come to greet you. What could happen? Perhaps they would be scared and wouldn't think that it is likely to fly in a metallic bird. You may offer them a ride, and they could choose to run from you. People can refuse or resist new ideas, even if they are good ideas.

Your subconscious (mind-body) uses the combo of whatever you want (inspiration), what you believe, and what you expect as a blueprint for action. The results are achieved by your mind-body (unconscious), instead of by thinking or studying. If someone reaches a cold surface, she believes is very hot, she can bring in a blister or burn response.

Conversely, a person touching a scorching surface, presuming it's cold, may not produce a wake response. People who walk across hot flashes while imagining they're cool may experience thermal injury (some minor overlaps around the bottoms of their toes). But their immune system does not respond with a burn (blistering, pain, etc.) because their minds notify their bodies of the best way to reply. Again, it is the alignment of all of those very Important ingredients that make this possible. That's the trick to success. Your whole body carries your beliefs; your beliefs direct your actions, which then sort your experience. Some describe this process as creating your accomplishment or generating your experience in life.

Within our culture, we see this clarified in the inspirational and positive psychological outlook literature. It might be known in many areas of metaphysics. It's also likely to return into the ancients and observe that's explained in the historical period's particulars.

A person much wiser than we are said, "It will be done telling you according to your perspective." In the present age of alcoholism and medicine, we call it self-hypnosis or mind-body medicine. There continue to be several scientific studies that show surprising effects for pain control, wound healing, bodily change, and much more health benefits than we believed possible.

Spiritual Awakening

Dr. Sebi believed that the way to live a truly spiritual life was to live in such a way that you are "cosmically connected" to everything. This means living in tune with the laws of nature, so that there is harmony in the world on all physical, mental, and spiritual levels. He also said that if people call themselves spiritual but are still eating ham and potatoes and other acidic foods, he cannot relate to that kind of spirituality. For Dr. Sebi, an essential part of the spiritual life is getting the right type of diet. Only when an individual is balanced within, and has a healthy body free of excess mucus, are they ready to attain more sensitive spiritual awareness levels. Dr. Sebi's diet and lifestyle could be seen as a new kind of spiritual awakening.

Chapter 2

THE ALKALINE DIET AND INTRACELLULAR CLEANSING

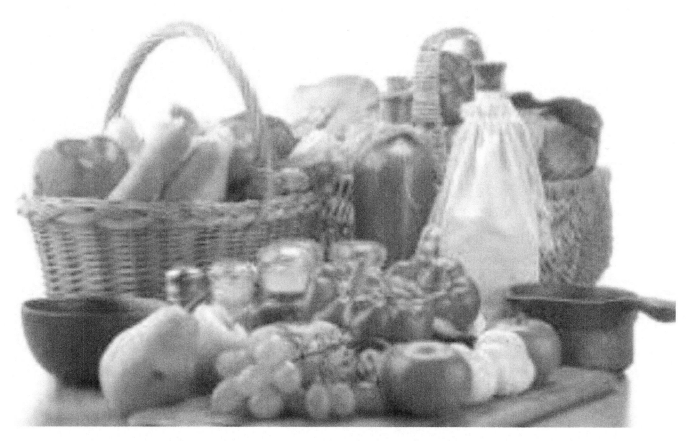

Dr. Sebi's prescribed process can help in cleansing and detoxifying the body. It is also known as intracellular cleanse. Juice cleansing or fasting can also help the same way but Dr. Sebi's methods usually focus on intracellular cleanse.

Intra-Cellular Cleansing Intracellular cleansing is the cleansing and rinsing of every cell. Dr. Sebi and USHA research institute advocates that to cleanse a body and its system, the cleansing on a cellular level corrects any imbalances or damages done over time.

The Accumulation of Stagnant Toxins

Dr. Sebi's diet is based on the idea that mucus is the source of our bodily ailments. If the mucus membrane has been damaged or compromised, this can result in all sorts of problems for the body. If excess mucus finds its way into our lungs, it will manifest in lung disease. If there is an excess of mucus in the stomach, it will display as stomach problems. Excess mucus can even result in forms of cancer for the afflicted organ. For this reason, Dr. Sebi described mucus as a stagnant toxin.

According to Dr. Sebi, an overly acidic diet can excess the stagnant toxin known as mucus. For example, foods high in starch are prime culprits. Animal products are another example. High acidity can lead to inflammation, which then compromises the mucus membrane and results in excess mucus disturbing other bodily organs.

How Do We Get Sick?

Here is one example of the process, laid out from start to finish. You eat a type of food that is considered too acidic (Dr. Sebi would describe it as "unnatural," which will be explained more fully in chapter 8). This food harms your mucus membrane, causing an excess amount of mucus to pass over into other organs of the body. When too much mucus has accumulated in a particular organ such as the lungs, it manifests in that organ's sickness.

This is in stark contrast to what Dr. Sebi describes as "Western medical research," as it rejects the idea that bacteria, germs, and viruses cause sickness. Dr. Sebi proposes that it is not germs that make us unwell, but an excess of mucus spread throughout the body.

Cleansing of the Organs

Cleansing at the cellular level also cleans body organs. Let's understand these processes in more detail.

The Colon

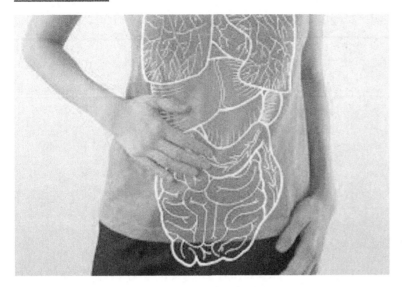

The colon is the most critical organ in the body, and it must be cleansed by detoxifying to reverse any possible diseases. Your colon is essential for your good health. It contains good bacteria and healthy flora which helps in the digestion and toxin removal from the body.

The Liver

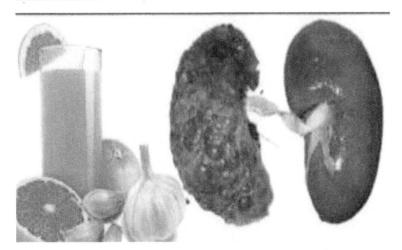

Your liver is a vital organ that supports most of the organs in your body. The liver helps in digestion by producing the essential biochemicals in the body. It also helps synthesize proteins, convert poisonous ammonia to urea, produce hormones, and detoxify the body's fluids by changing the composition of toxic substances.

The Lungs

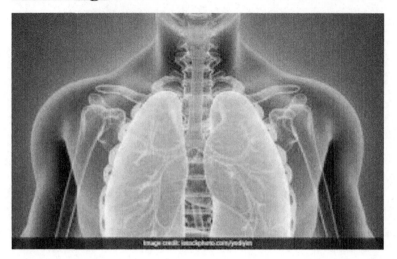

Lungs help in extracting oxygen from the air you breathe. This oxygen is then transferred into your bloodstream and exchanged with carbon dioxide released from the bloodstream back into the atmosphere.

However, lungs can also become overburdened with excessive internal pollution which can impair their functions.

The Lymphatic System

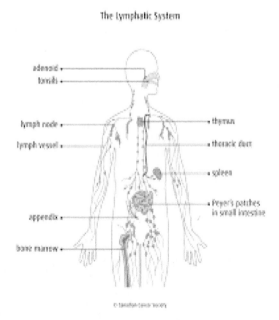

The lymphatic system is a complex network of lymphatic vessels that carry a fluid called lymph around the body. It also transports fats, proteins, and other substances to the blood system. The lymphatic system works as an immune system defense.

The Skin

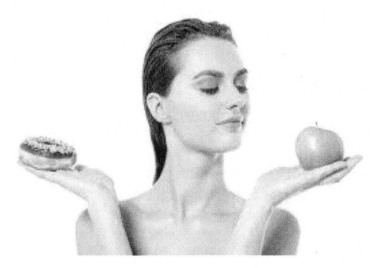

Your skin is the largest organ that is responsible for eliminating toxins from your body.

Skin is made up of two layers: the outer layer epidermis which acts as a waterproof barrier and no blood vessels.

How to Carry Out an Intra-Cellular Cleanse

Before you try to cleanse your systems, it is essential to understand the right food concept. Are you putting the right things into your body? You cannot expect a good cleansing process involving pH or alkalinity if your diet is very acidic.

These starter guides will help you to understand some tips and recipes regarding the cleansing process.

Dr. Sebi's Cleansing Compounds

If you have learned to eat or drink under control and feel that you are ready to follow Dr. Sebi's diet, you can consider the following compounds:

Chelation2

This compound increases bowels' movements and helps remove toxins from the body, like acid or mucus.

Viento

Viento works as an energizer, cleanser, and revitalizer.

Bio Ferro

Bio Ferro is a potent and effective blood purifier.

Can I Make My Compounds?

Dr. Sebi's compounds may be expensive for some people and they may try to make them at home. It is possible if you have done the right research and know every minute details of these compounds' composition.

However, it should be remembered that if you try to create them without proper understanding, you may not get precisely what Dr. Sebi prescribed.

Chapter 3

EXCESSIVE MUCUS IN THE BODY

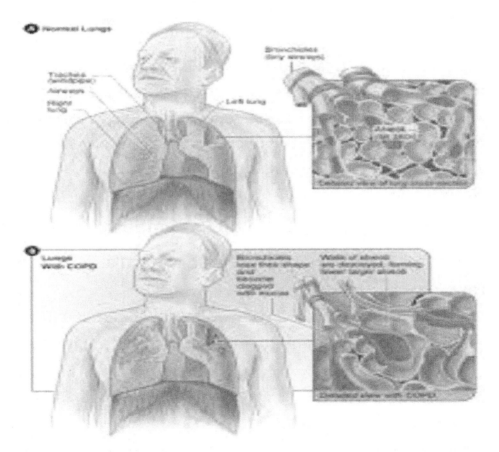

According to Dr. Sebi, mucus and acidity cause disease, and eating certain kinds of food and abstaining from others could lead to an alkaline state. This reduces the disease's risk and effects through the body's detoxification since illness cannot exist in an alkaline environment. So, he designed his 'African Bio-Mineral Theory' for anyone who desires to improve their health in general and cure or prevent disease without Western medicine. The goal of the 'African Bio-Mineral Therapy

Program' is to uncover the symptoms and examine and identify the disease's cause, which is mucus. Where there is accumulated mucus in the body, this place is linked to a disease manifestation. Even though the 'African Bio-Mineral Therapy Program' was designed to extract Mucus from the body, it can also serve as a cleansing and nourishing agent to the whole bodily system. This is what makes this therapeutic program unique.

Fourteen days after initially taken, these therapeutic compound cleansing properties are still being released into the body since the herbs used have a natural origin. With this approach, there has been a successful reversing of pathologies. Strict compliance with Dr. Sebi's nutritional guidelines is essential when undergoing the 'African Bio-Mineral Therapy Program.' The body will experience the best environment for maximum health because the herbal compound is synchronized with the outlined nutritional guidelines.

This diet focuses on natural, alkaline, plant-based foods and herbs, which involves consuming a certain amount of approved food with many supplements while staying away from hybrid, acidic foods that can damage the cell. Also, while following the diet, herbs are taken to nourish the cell, help cleanse the body, and heal those who participate in the program who have been on a horrible diet for years.

Dr. Sebi was a vegan and as such the diet's composition is a list of:

- Vegetables which includes avocado, kale, wild arugula, and bell peppers,
- Grains including wild rice, quinoa, rye, and spelled,
- Fruits which includes bananas, Seville orange, dates, and apples,
- Seeds and nuts including walnuts, raw sesame seeds, and hemp and tahini butter,
- Herbal teas which include, fennel, ginger varieties, and chamomile,
- Natural sweeteners, which include date sugar and agave syrup,
- Spices which includes powdered seaweed and cayenne and,
- Oil, including coconut, hempseed, olive, and avocado oils. Olive oil and coconut oil should not be used for cooking, as advised by the diet. This diet must be followed through if one intends to experience the body healing itself.

According to Dr. Sebi, there are six food categories: live, raw, dead, hybrid, genetically modified food, and drugs. Dr. Sebi believes live and raw foods are for the "healing of the nation" and are considered to be "electric foods" for the cell since they are of alkaline origin, and they help heal the body from adverse effects that acidic food has produced. While genetically modified food, hybrid, and drug-food, whether seedless fruits, weather-resistant crops like corn, or anything with added minerals or vitamins, should be avoided. Food like meat, poultry, and seafood, products containing yeast, sugar, alcohol, iodized salt, or anything fried that is acidic should also be avoided because they negatively affect the body.

For the individual that enjoys eating acidic food, following a raw diet mostly can seem unpalatable. You get used to it since your goal is to flush your toxins cells, which leads to the cure of the disease.

Dr. Sebi recommended some of his products for the cure of the herpes virus. The product names are Bromide Plus Powder, Iron Plus, and Bio Ferro. You can use these products by following the instructions written on them by Dr. Sebi. He also recommended certain herbs you can prepare yourself at home if you cannot buy the product.

Below are the main ingredients contained in Dr. Sebi's herpes products:

- AHP Zinc Powder
- Triphala
- Pure extract giloy tablets
- Punarnavadi Mandoor
- AHP Silver Powder

Detailed Analysis of the Elements

AHP Zinc Powder

The term AHP stands for ayurvedically herbs purified. The purification of zinc is done with decoctions of natural herbs such as Aloe Vera to produce AHP zinc powder. AHP zinc powder has a better benefit than the usual zinc tablets you consume. It is prepared from naturally occurring zinc, making it very easy for your body to absorb.

AHP zinc powder also has the main qualities of some of the herbs used in preparing it. Modern medicine also acknowledges the importance of zinc for herpes treatment, but it is better to use it instead of zinc tablets. This powder is safer and more effective in treating herpes.

Triphala

Triphala contains three outstanding herbal combinations. The three herbs that make up Triphala are amla, bibhitaki, and haritaki. These three herbs have not only been acknowledged for their potency by Dr. Sebi, but other medical experts have conducted research on these three great herbs and praised its efficacy.

This combination is the right one that can be taken by healthy persons and people infected with the herpes virus. This herbal combination can clean the unwanted materials and toxins in your body and help purify your blood and many organs in your body. Dr. Sebi didn't only administer this combination to his patients but also took daily optimal health and longevity.

Pure Extract Giloy Tablets

Pure extract giloy tablets are produced manually from the extracts of the best quality giloy. Giloy is the perfect herb to improve your immunity and fight sexually transmitted diseases (STDs).

Dr. Sebi himself was a big fan of Giloy, and now, modern medical experts have accepted that it can help your body fight off many diseases and improve health.

Punarnavadi Mandoor

Punarnavadi mandoor is not a purified herbal mineral, but a healthy herbomineral created from the combination of herbs and minerals. Punarnavadi mandoor is an extraordinary combination of beneficial minerals such as calcium, iron, and great herbs such as shunting, punarnava, alma, etc.

This herb mineral combination works perfectly on the liver and helps to eliminate toxins in the liver. Dr. Sebi administered this herb mineral combination to many of his patients, and the reason for this is that the liver's function was disrupted during infection. Punarnavadi Mandoor is the perfect option to bring the liver function back to normal.

AHP Silver Powder

Ayurvedically herbs purified (AHP) is a process that involves purifying various minerals in herbal decoctions making them useful for medication. AHP ensures that the minerals maintain their excellent abilities and absorb the herbs' nutrition and qualities, which they are purified into. AHP powder is beneficial to your health, especially your nervous system. Dr. Sebi administered AHP silver powder to several of his patients with herpes, and the results were always right.

What makes AHP silver powder effective for herpes is that it works on your neurons. This is the very place where the herpes virus resides, using your body as their home and hiding place. This powder works by sending silver nanoparticles into your neurons to eliminate and flush out the herpes virus in your neurons.

Chapter 4

ELECTRIC FOOD AND FORESTS

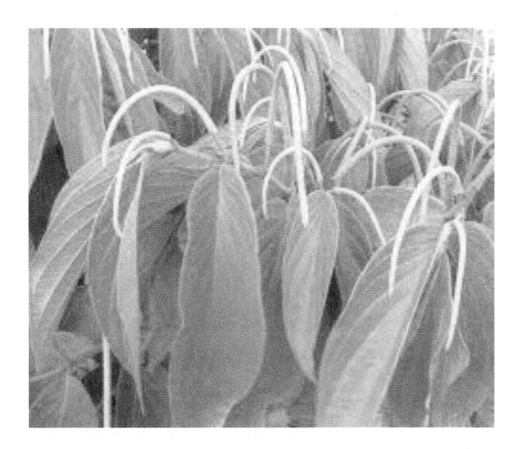

Cordoncillo Negro

Cordoncillo Negro is a tropical alkaline flowering plant from the family of 'Piperaceae'. This seed-producing plant contains compounds like beta-caryophyllene, ocimene, and dillapiole which makes it a beneficial herb to treat various health disorders and as an antiseptic, to stop hemorrhages, treatment of ulcers, genitals and urinary organs, etc.

The Benefits of Consuming Cordoncillo Negro

- The benefits of consuming Cordoncillo Negro include:
- It helps to stop bleeding and heals wounds with its anti-septic properties.
- It helps to treat and prevent infections that are caused by bacteria and viruses.
- It helps to treat and prevent ulcers through its anti-septic properties.
- It helps to eliminate and prevent the growth of viruses and bacteria.
- It helps to expel gas and to remove mucus from the body and stop spewing.
- It helps treat and prevent sexually transmitted diseases (STD) such as gonorrhea, syphilis, herpes, etc.
- It enhances digestion and boosts digestive health, treats and prevents digestive disorders like dyspepsia and diarrhea, etc.
- It helps to enhance the health of the kidney and liver and inhibit the development of kidney stones.

Side Effects of Consuming Cordoncillo Negro

Till at the time of writing this book, there are no side effects that have been attributed to consuming Cordoncillo Negro.

What Precautions Should Be Taken Before Using Cordoncillo Negro?

There are no precautions to be noted because this herb is 100% safe for all to consume.

What Are the Medications That Interacts with Cordoncillo Negro?

There are no medications that interact with Cordoncillo Negro.

What Is the Dosage and How is Cordoncillo Negro Tea Prepared?

For the dosage and how to prepare Cordoncillo Negro tea, kindly take the following steps:

1. Harvest some fresh leaves of Cordoncillo Negro, wash, and dried it until it is dried.
2. Once it is dried, chopped or pound it into smaller pieces. You can order it online and it will come dried and chopped.
3. Boil 8-10ounce of water.

4. Measure 1teaspoon of Cordoncillo Negro and pour it into your teacup or mug.
5. Pour the boiling water in the cup or mug where the Cordoncillo Negro is and cover for 10-15 minutes to steep.
6. Allow it to get cold and strain it. You are done!
7. For the dosage, consume 1 cup (8ounce) of the Cordoncillo Negro tea 2-3 times daily.

Contribo

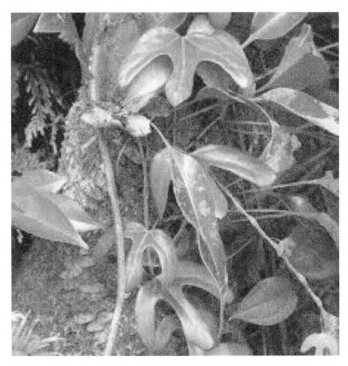

Contribo is a vine plant from the family of Aristolochiaceae. Dr. Sebi recommends as a revitalizing herb because of its potency in rejuvenating the loss of energy that the body must have lost due to the disease, enrich mood, fight fatigue, boost appetite, etc.

What Are the Benefits of Consuming Contribo?

The benefits of consuming Contribo are:

- It helps to boost energy and stamina levels.
- It helps to enrich mood and relieve fatigue and depression.
- It helps to enhance and boost the circulatory system and also, increase appetite.

- It helps to combat delayed menstruation and fast track it.
- It helps enhance the health of the digestive system and gallbladder and also relieves constipation.
- It helps to treat and prevent kidney disorder, dissolves kidney stones, and enhances kidney's health.
- It helps to treat and dissolves bladder stones and also, relieve uterine complaints.
- It helps to boost the immune defense system and also, calm and heal the immune system.
- It helps treat and prevent various diseases such as flu, stomach irritation, indigestion, colds, non-insulin-dependent diabetes, etc.

What Are the Side Effects of Consuming Contribo?

Till at the time of writing this book, there are no side effects that have been attributed to the use or consumption of contribo.

What Precautions Should Be Taken Before Consuming Contribo?

The precautions that should be taken are:

- Because there is not much information on whether this herb is harmful to pregnant or breastfeeding mothers, I advise that they avoid this herb.
- If you have or have ever suffered from any kidney disorder, consult with your doctor before consuming this herb
- You shouldn't use this herb for long because of the aristolochic acid that it contains that can damage human health in the long run.

What Are the Medications That Interact with Contribo?

Till at the time of writing this book, there are no medications that interact with Contribo.

What Is the Dosage and Should Contribo Tea or Infusion Be Prepared?

1. For the dosage and how to prepare Contribo tea or infusion, kindly take the steps below:
2. Harvest some fresh vine of contribo, wash it, and dry it.

3. Once it is dried, chop it into smaller pieces or order it online and it will come dried and chopped.
4. Measure 1-2 teaspoon of contribo and add it to your saucepan.
5. Pour 8-16 ounce of water and add it to the saucepan where the contribo vine is.
6. Boil the mixture for 10-15 minutes.
7. After boiling it, strain it, you are done!
8. For the dosage, take 1-2cups of contribo tea 2 times per day (preferably, morning and night).
9. Alternatively, if you have the fresh vine, wash it and soak it in boiling water 24 hours.
10. For the dosage, ½ cups per week.

Pavana

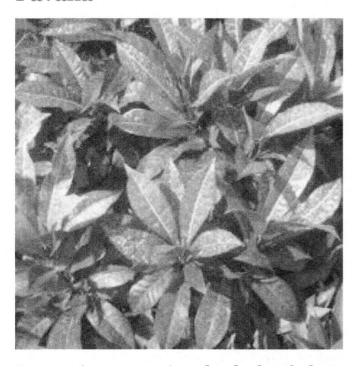

Pavana is a purgative shrub that belongs to the family of the Euphorbiaceae. Dr. Sebi recommended this herb as his favorite herbs that have the potency to make you spew, a tool that helps to purge the body.

<u>What Are the Benefits of Consuming Pavana?</u>

- The benefits of consuming Pavana include:
- It helps to destroy cancerous cells and prevent the cells from mutating.

- It helps to treat and prevent dysentery and constipation
- It helps to treat and prevent gallbladder disorder and dissolves gallbladder stone.
- It helps to soothe digestive problems or disorders.
- It helps to unblock blocked intestines
- It helps to treat various fevers such as malaria fever
- It helps to treat colitis, gout, and relieve joint (rheumatism) pain.
- It helps to treat, calm, and boost the health of the nerves (neuralgia) pain.
- It helps to treat skin disorders like eczema.
- It helps to boost the health of the bronchial tubes and treat bronchitis.

What Are the Side Effects of Consuming Pavana?

The side effects that you can suffer from consuming Pavana are:

- It can lead to death (a few drops of its oil taking by mouth).
- Spewing
- Diarrhea
- Burning sensation (possibly in the mouth and throat)
- Dizziness

What Precautions Should Be Taken Before Consuming Pavana?

Pavana is not safe for anyone but if you must consume it, consult with your doctor. It can also lead to miscarriage for pregnant women.

What Is the Dosage and How Should Pavana Tea or Infusion Be Prepared?

Please if you order for the herb online, follow the prescribed dosage on the package label and ensure you consult your doctor before using this herb.

Kalawalla

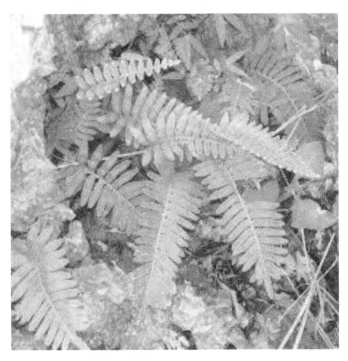

Kalawalla is a type of fern that is a nonflowering vascular plant belonging to the Pteridophyta botanical family.

Because of the effectiveness of Kalawalla on the treatment of skin disorders such as vitiligo, treating multiple sclerosis, boosting the immune defense system, neutralizing free radicals and protecting DNA cells, eliminating toxins from the body, helping the body to heal and recover quickly, etc. Dr. Sebi recommended Kalawalla as a revitalization herb to help the body heal quickly.

What Are the Benefits of Consuming Kalawalla?

The benefits of consuming Kalawalla are:

- It helps treat and prevent inflammation and skin allergies like sunburn, eczema, psoriasis, redness of the skin, etc.
- It helps to protect DNA cells from damage that is caused by free radicals.
- It helps to boost, regulate and balance the immune defense system.
- It helps to treat and prevent inflammatory disorders like inflamed skin, hives, rashes, etc.
- It helps to enrich overall mood, relief, and treat anxiety and depression.
- It helps to boost energy and fight against fatigue and numbness.

- It helps treat brain disorders such as Alzheimer's and dementia, paranoid, Parkinson's, etc.
- It helps to treat thyroid disorder like Grave's disease, Hashimoto's disease, etc.
- It helps to treat diabetes by lowering blood sugar levels.
- It helps treat and prevent other health disorders like, scleroderma, lupus, Crohn's disease, arthritis, hemolytic anemia, etc.

What Are the Side Effects of Using Kalawalla?

When writing this book, no side effect is attributed to Kalawalla herb's consumption.

What Precautions Should Be Taken Before Consuming Kalawalla?

Because there is not enough information to ascertain whether this herb is harmful to pregnant and breastfeeding mothers, I advise them to avoid using this herb.

What Are the Medications That Interact with Kalawalla?

Kalawalla interacts with heart medication. Such medications include:

- Digitalis
- Bisoprolol (Zebeta)
- Atenolol (Tenormin)
- Bisoprolol/hydrochlorothiazide (Ziac)
- Propranolol (Inderal)
- Metoprolol (Lopressor/Toprol XL)
- Acebutolol (Sectral)
- Nadolol (Corgard)
- Betaxolol (Kerlone) etc.

What Is the Dosage and How Should Kalawalla Tea Be Prepared?

For the dosage and how to prepare Kalawalla tea, kindly take the following steps:

1. Harvest some fresh leaves of Kalawalla plant and wash it, dried it and if it is dried, pound it.
2. Alternatively, you can place an order online and it will come dried and pound.

3. Measure 1teaspoon of the pounded Kalawalla leaves and add it to your teacup or mug.
4. Boil 8 ounce of water and pour it into the cup/mug with the Kalawalla leaves.
5. Cover it and allow it to steep for 15-20minutes and step it down.
6. Strain it. You are done!
7. For the dosage, take 1cup (8ounce) of Kalawalla tea 1-3 times daily.

Sea Moss

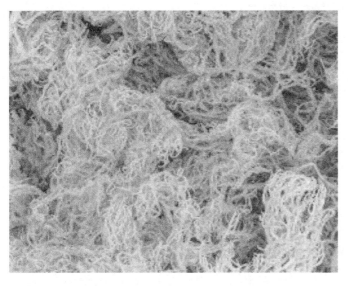

Irish Sea Moss is red algae that belongs to the family of Florideophytes that grows on the rocky parts of the Atlantic coast of various countries like the British Isles, Ireland, Jamaica, Scotland, etc. One amazing fact about this herb that makes Dr. Sebi recommend it for cleansing and revitalizing the body system is that it contains about 92 out of the 102 minerals that the body needs to be healthy. Some of the minerals that it contains are iodine, selenium, calcium, bromine, zinc, iron, phosphorus, potassium, etc.

What Are the Benefits of Consuming Irish Sea Moss?

The benefits of consuming Irish Sea Moss are:

- It helps to heal and boost the immune defense system.
- It helps to treat and prevent hyperthyroidism and boost the functionalities and health of the thyroid gland.
- It helps to soothe joint pain and swelling of the joint and treat arthritis.
- It helps to enrich overall mood and reduce fussiness.
- It helps to combat infections caused by viruses and bacteria.

- It helps to treat and prevent digestive and respiratory tract disorders
- It helps to treat and prevent various skin disorders like acne, skin wrinkling, and alleviates inflammation.

What Are the Side Effects of Consuming Irish Sea Moss?

The side effects of consuming Irish Sea moss are:

- Spewing
- Burning sensation or itching (mouth and throat)
- Fever
- Stomach irritation
- Nausea

What Precautions Should Be Taken Before Consuming Irish Sea Moss?

The precautions that should be taken are:

- Because of how rich Irish Sea moss is with iron, it can trigger hypothyroidism for people suffering from Hashimoto's disease.
- Stop using the herb if you notice any allergic reaction.

What Is the Dosage and How Should Irish Sea Moss Tea Be Prepared?

For the dosage and how to prepare Irish Sea Moss tea, kindly take the steps below:

1. Measure and boil 1cups (8ounce) of water in a ceramic pot.
2. Once the water is boiled, measure 2-3 tablespoon of Irish Sea moss gel (or 1teaspoon for the powdery form) and add it to the boiling water.
3. Allow the Irish Sea moss for 10-15 minutes to dissolve completely.
4. You are done! For the dosage, take 1cup (8ounce) of Irish Sea moss tea daily in the morning.

Sarsaparilla

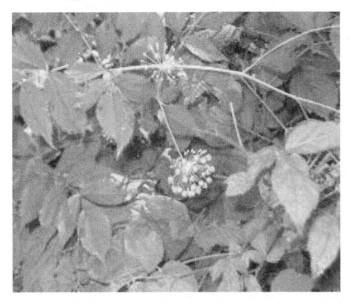

Sarsaparilla is a tropical wood climbing vine that belongs to the genus Smilax family. It is very rich with iron, calcium, phosphate, sarsaponin steroid, flavonoid, etc body needs to speed up the healing and recovery process. Late Dr. Sebi recommended sarsaparilla as a revitalizing herb because of its potency to fast track healing and recovery process.

What Are the Benefits of Consuming Sarsaparilla?

The benefits of consuming Sarsaparilla are:

- It binds the endotoxins responsible for the lesions in psoriasis patients and eliminates it from the body system.
- It helps treat and prevent health issues caused by inflammation like joint pain, swelling of any parts of the body, arthritis, rheumatoid, etc.
- It helps to soothe and heals sexually transmitted diseases such as syphilis, herpes, gonorrhea, etc.
- It helps to treat and prevent leprosy
- It helps to destroy and prevent cancerous cells from mutating.
- It helps to protect, and reverse damages done to the liver to function correctly.
- It helps to make the body absorb nutrients and other herbs quickly etc.

What Precautions Should Be Taken Before Consuming Sarsaparilla Root?

The precautions that should be taken are:

- Check your temperature if it's above 100, do not consume sarsaparilla.
- Since there is no information to know if this herb is harmful to pregnant or breast-feeding mothers, I advise that they stay off this herb.

What Are the Side Effects of Consuming Sarsaparilla Root?

Till at the time of writing this book, there are no side effects attributed to this herb's consumption. However, because of the 'saponins' that it contains, I advise you to consult your doctor before using this herb as saponins can cause stomach irritation.

What Is the Dosage and How Should Sarsaparilla Root Tea Be Prepared?

For the dosage and how to prepare sarsaparilla root tea, kindly take the following steps:

- Harvest some sarsaparilla plant roots and wash it under running water to remove all the dirt that accompanied it from the soil.
- After washing it, pill off the outer skin, chop it into smaller pieces, and dry it in a well-ventilated place (indoors) for at least seven days (ensure you turn the drying root daily for the 7 days until it is completely dried.)
- Once it is dried, store it in a paper bag or cardboard box. (Ensure you don't keep it in a plastic container as it will get mold).
- Measure 1teaspoon of the dried chopped Sarsaparilla root and add it to your saucepan and add 8 ounces of water. Boil it for 15-20minutes
- Strain it using a strainer. You are done!

For the dosage, consume 1cup (8ounce) 3 times daily.

Chapter 5

THE GUT-BRAIN CONNECTION

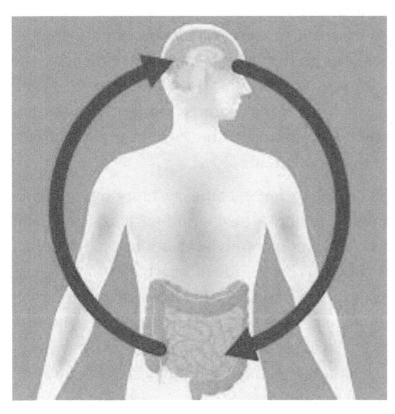

Our overall health is set through the filter of our perception. The power of thought-belief-placebo has been well-studied, documented, and repeated scientifically throughout history. "If we believe it, then we see it" is a concept that has been previously discussed. Still, many feel unable or unwilling to open their minds to information beyond their existing mindsets and beliefs—especially in this subject, for those uneducated in nutrition. Even for me, who has an abundance of nutritional education, it has been a long journey. The evidence now has mounted to an undeniable truth: there is a powerful gut-brain connection. The human gut microbiome is much more powerful and in control of our destiny, health, and wellness than we ever thought probable or possible.

Human culture has known for millennia that our gut and brain work together. Both our conscious and unconscious minds assess our environment, to "think things through." Often, the subconscious or unconscious mind is really "feeling things through," using our gut reactions or gut instincts first to assess the person or situation and then make a decision. For example, we sometimes know very quickly if we dislike or trust someone, want to see a person better, hire them, date them, or even marry them.

Recent medical research has dramatically expanded our knowledge of the concept of the gut-brain connection. We now know more about the fact that this connection works both ways. For example, the brain has a dramatic influence over the gut and the other way around. This was initially surprising to the medical community, which saw these as totally separate, with the brain being in charge.

Now, we know the gut has power over the brain and can cause havoc, if not nurtured properly. This is seen through the expanse of all sorts of human disease, which we now know starts in the gut and can cause everything from cravings to significant illnesses. These communications go through the nervous and endocrine systems. Stimulations are known to go both brain-to-gut and gut-to-brain. Nerves—primarily the Vagus nerve—provide a direct connection between the gut and brain. Also, chemical or hormonal stimulation from various organs affects communication—both ways—through the bloodstream.

In our human evolution, the body needed to favor some systems over others, during specific experiences. For example, we shut down some parts of the gut or the brain to allow another to take over the blood supply, our attention, and react immediately in crisis or emergency times. This is meant to be a good thing, imperative for our survival. However, in modern society, this unconscious reaction to stress creates a vicious cycle. Psychological stress can increase gut permeability and change the population of the gut bacteria. The imbalance is known as dysbiosis, which leads to increased leakiness of the tight junctions in the gut, ultimately leading to more significant inflammation.

Food, Mood, and Mental Health

Mental health has a long history of stigmatization in human society. Even though there has likely always been mental illness in all cultures, there have been varying degrees of acceptance and treatment. Some cultures forbid showing any weakness, especially regarding mental health concerns. Other cultures may sympathize, to a degree, but asking for help can be difficult, and finding it can be even more challenging. As a result, suicide statistics are at an all-time high. Anxiety and depression medications are often distributed to patients before any other option. Most often, in our western society, by the time a real problem in mental health is discovered or disclosed, it has grown beyond the point of an easy fix. Typically, medical doctors are involved in treatment and prescription drugs are the norm. This trend of using drugs for treating mental health has led to drug overuse and abuse. Addictions and side effects of medications are also the norm, with little change in the approach. However, these drugs do not make the problem go away, and often, the outcome is having to continue with the prescription for the rest of one's life.

Information on the connection of the gut and brain has been around for many years. It has gone in and out of favor over the last 100 years, since it was first published, causing a new wave of interest in this topic worldwide. Being an MD, with specialties in neurology and nutrition, and the mother of an autistic child, Dr. Natasha Campbell-McBride_was highly motivated to gather together the latest research of the time. Her connection between diet and brain development (with the backdrop of Autism and a mother's motivation) addressed this condition's considerable increase in various populations. Being so widespread, her mention of "doctors, biochemists, biologists, and simply intelligent human beings as parents, looking for solutions to their child's problems,"_banded organizations together and may just have been the seed which fueled the interest in the gut-brain connection and the study of the human gut microbiome.

Some of the most significant advances in the last few years in the connection between food and mood (our mental health) have occurred in the Food and Mood Centre research at Deakin University in Australia. Many studies_from the Food and Mood Centre—both complete and in-progress—point to the increasing evidence that food directly impacts mood and specific mental health issues. Food has sometimes been proven to be more impactful than current medications and certainly, much better than placebos. Food even changes our DNA! Not only does nutrition influence our physical and mental health, but it also has a direct connection to the health and wellbeing of our microbiota. The microbiota in our GI tract is now seen as a separate "organ," referred to as the "second brain," and has been and is being connected to many and perhaps even all human diseases.

Let's now look at where and how the gut-brain connection affects mental and physical health.

How the Gut-Brain Connection Affects Mental Health

Mental Illness and Healing

It is a well-known fact that the brain needs oxygen to function. According to Dr. Sebi's philosophy, an excessive amount of mucus can block the oxygen flow that the brain relies upon so urgently. Mucus that resides in the mind can eventually manifest as illness: "physical" illness and mental illness. Dementia, Parkinson's disease, Alzheimer's disease, and other neurological conditions can be blamed on excessive mucus in the brain, preventing oxygen from reaching it. As a result of the lack of oxygen, thought patterns begin to change and the body becomes distressed. A lack of iron in particular can be responsible for this diminished flow of oxygen to the brain. This is why Dr. Debi recommends alkalized foods rather than the acidic foods that cause the build-up of excessive mucus in the first place. Mental health conditions such as anxiety and depression have a similar cause.

Anxiety and Depression

It is common to suffer from both anxiety and depression at the same time, but not always. Sometimes, persistent anxiety is what leads to depressive symptoms. The chief difference between the two is that anxiety is characterized by fear, apprehension, nervous thoughts, and exaggerated worries about the future. Depression doesn't entail such concern. Depression revolves around a sense of hopelessness—the sky has already fallen, life is bad, and nothing can go right.

Anxiety and depression are often cached together because they are related psychologically and have many similar physical symptoms (negative thinking, headaches, pain, nausea, and GI problems). Depression and anxiety both suffer disruption of the gut microbiota. Numerous studies have found the same kinds of features in those with anxiety disorder as in those with depression:

While the research is still in its infancy, it has become clear that anxiety disorders and depression are caused by a combination of factors that most definitely include the state and function of the gut and its inhabitants. Further studies recognized that it was not enough to feed the subjects just probiotics, but the probiotics must be provided. Adding food for the "good bacteria" in probiotic or specific fiber resulted in good psychological changes. The underlying theory was that if you're anxious to begin with, you'll be more reactive to negativity as well as emotionally-charged images and/or words. Subjects who increased their consumption of prebiotics foods (high fiber) and paid more attention to positive information had less anxiety with negative stimuli and lower cortisol levels. These results are similar to individuals on antidepressants. Other research relates the microbiota of the intestine with diseases of the nervous system and its possible treatment through the use of good bacteria. This is excellent news for those wanting to solve the original problems rather than just treating symptoms with pharmaceuticals.

Immunity

It has been mentioned before that immunity is directly connected to the gut microbiota's inoculation through a normal, healthy, timely, natural birth. When a baby passes through the vaginal canal, the mother's bacterial culture's health implants her baby's lifelong health while passing through. If born via a Caesarian section, the baby becomes inoculated with cells from the operating room, including skin and other cells from the surgical team, the mother, father, and others in the scrubbed room. This inoculation prepares the infant's entire digestive system to have the ability to digest breast milk. The breast milk ingredients then prepare the gut for other ingested foods, as child development occurs. When babies are born without this preparation for the child's life, it starts a cascade of events that may incur infections (such as throat or ear infections), precipitating antibiotics' use and overuse. This launch is anything but healthy for the child's life and sets patterns that can last a lifetime.

Studies have shown that babies born by C-section have a higher incidence of immunity problems, develop more diseases and allergies, and are more prone to obesity later in life. The cause appears to be the lack of a proper transfer of the gut microbiota. This research also includes the discovery of the inclusion of foodstuffs in breast milk that have nothing to do with the baby's feeding. Infants cannot digest it. This discovery has set a myriad of assumptions about the meaning of health for infants. This revelation shocked the medical community and emphasized the importance of having a vaginal birth and successful breastfeeding. We knew it was necessary, but we now know how important it is. This is the first real evidence that these natural processes are essential for human growth and development and a healthy life after that. There is also increasing evidence that the timing of gestation accompanies a timing of vaginal microbiome development so that both come together to be of the best benefit for the newborn's success.

Chapter 6

FASTING

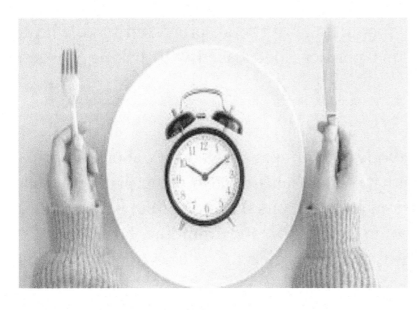

There are various detoxification types, but I will center on fasting, which is the one approved by the late Dr. Sebi. Under the fasting method of detoxification, there are various types of fasting which include:

Dry fasting: Under this fasting type, you will abstain from food, water, juice, anything eatable or drinkable.

Liquid fasting: Under this fasting type, you can abstain from anything solid and consume only liquids like juice and any other liquid stuff without alcohol.

Water fasting: Under this type of fasting, you can abstain from anything solid, juice, smoothies, etc., and consume only water.

Fruit fasting: Under this type of fasting, you can avoid anything solid but survive mainly on fruit.

Raw food fasting: Under this fasting type, you can abstain entirely from cooked food and survive mainly on veggies and fruit.

Smoothie fasting: Smoothie fasting is just like fruit fasting, the only difference is that under smoothie fasting, the fruit will be blended, and you will also consume blended veggies.

Bear in mind that Dr. Sebi approved 12 days fast with alkaline herbs, sea moss, spring water, and alkaline juice which must be made with fruit in Dr. Sebi's nutritional guide list.

Bad Habits

These are some bad habits of dieting:

Eating the Wrong Foods

Eating seedless fruits, canned vegetables, canned fruits, dairy, eggs, fish, poultry, red meat, soy products, take away food, restaurant food, processed food, wheat, fortified foods, sugar, alcohol, baking powder, food baked with baking powder, yeast, and food risen with yeast.

Drinking the Wrong Drinks

Dr. Sebi, just like health organizations, encourages drinking a gallon of spring water daily so that the diet is effective. Water helps remove waste products from the body, assist in nutrient absorption, and cushions the joints. Many of Dr. Sebi's approved herbs increase urination to remove toxins from the body and are diuretics. Therefore, your body will require water to replace the ones being excreted.

Glucose Dependency

Whenever you eat food, your body gets some blood glucose which is the main source of energy, and the insulin hormone produced by the pancreas ensures the blood glucose gets into the cells to be used as energy. Most cases of diabetes are because their pancreas does not produce a sufficient amount of insulin or their body does not use insulin well and the blood sugar remains in their blood without reaching the cells to be used as energy. Thus, the blood sugar level becomes too high.

According to Dr. Sebi, diabetes is usually caused by the blockage of the pancreatic duct caused by the mucus membrane having been compromised (broken) in the pancreatic duct and won't produce enough insulin hormone to break down sugar into energy.

Chapter 7

HOW TO PURIFY THE LIVER, GUT, AND INTESTINE

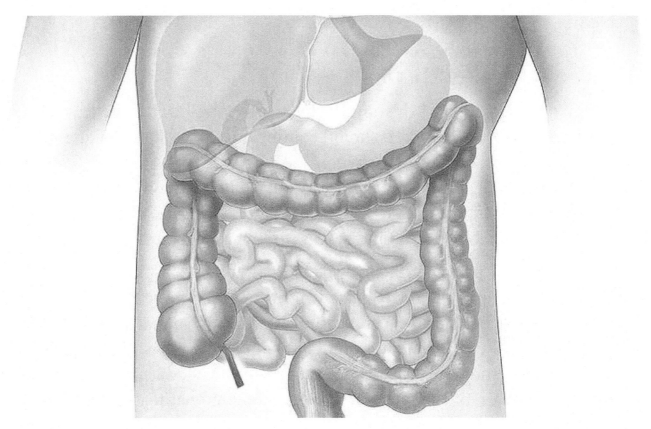

Different liver weight control plans are everywhere. One can find an eating routine of this nature online adequately. A couple of nourishments simply last several days while others keep going up to three weeks. Water also plays a critical role in any liver detox diet. A person who is going on such an eating regimen should drink eight cups of water each day to be powerful. Low-quality foods, processed foods, alcohol, coffee, and medications must be given up while going on a liver detox diet.

Purification of the Body

According to Dr. Sebi's diet, natural botanical remedies must be used consistently to purify the body and restore it to its natural alkaline state. After years of erosion and damage to the bodily organs, Dr. Sebi's 'African bio-mineral balance' restores and rejuvenates the body, replacing depleted minerals. When all of the excessive and stagnant toxins are removed from the skin, kidneys, liver, gallbladder, colon, and lymph glands, the body will start to heal. The colon is especially important, and the body cannot be rid of disease until the colon is first purified of all excess mucus.

Once every cell in the body is purified, the body can rejuvenate, and true health will be restored. Dr. Sebi recommends the following detox plan to purify the body properly:

The Seven Day Liver Detox Diet Plan

Day 1-Day 3: This period of this diet includes drinking just fluids. An individual who sets out on this specific diet; should confine oneself to just drinking new lime squeeze and water loads. This stage is one of the most troublesome, as an individual is fundamentally fasting and will feel feeble and tired. On the off chance that the person wants, one can do some light exercise while on this liver detox diet. It is important to enable a lot of time to rest and not exaggerate.

Day 4 - Day 6: This period of the liver detox diet is a lot simpler to deal with. An individual can eat every homemade food grown from the ground. Entire grain nourishments and bubbled vegetables are additionally permitted. Nonetheless, while an individual can eat certain nourishments at this phase of the detox diet, the person in question will likewise need to keep drinking many fluids. Fluids allowed at this phase of the menu are juices, home-grown teas, and handcrafted soil juice products.

Day 7: One can eat similar nourishments that are taken into account days 4 - 6. One can likewise steam their vegetables as opposed to eating them either crude or bubbled. Herbs that are prescribed for this phase of the diet are Rosemary and Dandelion.

While going on a liver detox diet is an extraordinary method to enable the liver to wipe out poisons from the framework, it can have negative symptoms. A separate ought to counsel their PCP before setting out on this kind of purging. For example, a person who encountered indications, retching, and agony should promptly stop the diet and look for medicinal assistance.

The Most Effective Method to Cleanse Your Liver

There are numerous ways on the most proficient method to detox your body, and despite the truth that it very well may be exceptionally testing, it isn't inconceivable. Vital nourishment for the liver detox is as of now referenced previously. Make sure to remember that nourishment for the day by day diet and drink loads of water each day. Liver detox is an incredible method to filter the liver from every one of the body's poisons. If the liver gets exhausted and an individual neglects to detox his/her liver, the liver may all of a sudden separate and discharge a pool of smelling salts into the blood. This is hazardous and can prompt severe harm to the sensory system, liver, mind, and kidneys. Likewise, the body may discharge lactic acid, causing constant weariness, hurting muscles, cerebral pain, tension, alarm assaults, and hypertension.

Step-by-Step Instructions to Start a Liver Detox Diet

A healthy liver can be acquired with the best possible measure of the correct sort of diet. The liver purging diet is presently a need in the general public. Most nourishment that individuals eat nowadays contains additives and fake added substances significant for long stockpiling periods yet destructive for our liver. To have a productive and successful liver purging diet, you should begin the correct way. So how are we going to start our liver purging food?

Before beginning a liver detoxification diet, make a list on the side effects (hypersensitivities, stench, nervousness, asthma, swelling, hypertension, low blood method, cold feet and hands, desires, stoppage, misery, looseness of the bowels, dry hair, dry skin, low energy, unpredictable glucose, weight addition, peevishness, and others) that you are presently encountering. Screen your body once per month to note if your body has come back to its best condition. It is additionally useful to make a rundown of nourishment that you expend to figure out what food should be dispensed with and what is to be kept up.

Seven days before the beginning of executing your liver purifying diet, you should quit smoking and drinking mixed drinks to avert over-burdening the liver that may cause trouble in wiping out harmful squanders that have gathered in our body. Additionally, have a healthy diet by taking up crisp products of the soil and reducing nourishments with a high measure of additives and other prepared food sources. Recollect that enormous numbers of the nourishments we expend every day contain unnatural poisons, for example, cancer-causing agents, anti-infection agents, pesticides, hormone medications, and fake sugars that may harm our liver.

Body condition is fundamental before a liver purging detox. Significantly, your body is decidedly ready to take a detox since you won't be permitted to devour healthy nourishments during a detox diet. It is also prudent to examine the liver detox plan with your doctor to evade different inconveniences to happen. Legitimate exercise will likewise have a molded body when a detox diet.

Light fasting seven days before your purging diet can be beneficial. The light diet contains heaps of water, crisp organic product juices, raw vegetables, and new natural products. New nourishments include more compounds that are fundamental in your liver purging diet. It additionally makes sure to eat at the correct time to abstain from overemphasizing your liver during the body melding. When your body is adapted, the danger of encountering undesirable reactions will be diminished.

Body detoxification can be begun with lessening your utilization of nourishments with a high amount of poisons, such as prepared food sources, liquor, artificial sugar, and espresso, and increment your measure of admission of new leafy foods.

The Importance of the Liver's Health in Weight Management

How significant is it to have a healthy liver when following a weight loss program?

Non-alcoholic fatty liver disease is, at present, the most widely recognized liver disease around the world. All non-alcoholic greasy liver disease phases are presently accepted because of insulin obstruction, a condition intently connected with heftiness.

Tests show that in individuals with liver issues, the higher an individual's BMI (Body Mass Index), the more prominent the liver harm. Perhaps the best worry in this nation is obesity in children. Furthermore, wouldn't you know it, so is youth NAFLD (Non-alcoholic Fatty Liver Disease)?

Losing excess weight is the foundation of the treatment of non-alcoholic greasy liver disease. There are meds that specialists can use to treat NAFLD; however, shedding pounds through diet and exercise is as yet the absolute best treatment. Nonetheless, this might be quite difficult. We live in a general public where high-fat, high carbohydrate, unhealthy nourishments are the standard, and exercise is an exertion. Diabetes is a scourge, and it is evaluated that 90% of individuals with Type 2 diabetes have greasy liver disease.

Insulin Resistance is the most significant contributing component of stoutness. Stomach fat is the snitch story indication of Insulin Resistance. How would you look? You may require some assistance, yet diabetes and weight increase can be overseen. Finally, advancing healthy dietary patterns and a functioning way of life, particularly in children, will most completely counteract NAFLD (greasy liver disease) and Type 2 diabetes.

Greasy liver in itself is nothing to stress over and will vanish with loss of weight. The ideal test approach is a straightforward blood test to check whether liver chemicals come back to ordinary after weight loss. If they do, you can be quite well sure NAFLD (non-alcoholic greasy liver disease) was the issue. In any case, to be satisfied, solitary a liver biopsy can tell, which is costly and nosy, and for the most part, not worth the dangers.

Artichoke and Sarsaparilla are an incredible mix of liver health. Artichoke improves liver capacity, including bile generation for fat digestion; Increases the excellent HDL cholesterol; Lowers raised blood lipids, cholesterol, and triglycerides; and Detoxes the liver and different organs of the body.

Sarsaparilla cleanses the blood, helps in bladder health and hormone balance in the two people. Look at it. It is anything but a regular thing. On more than one occasion per year should keep most everyone's liver running right, particularly on the off chance that they are eating right and practicing and not manhandling their liver with broad liquor utilization.

Control your weight and secure your liver simultaneously. Your health may rely upon it. If you or somebody realize they have excessive tummy fat, truly consider

NAFLD. This impacts children, just as grown-ups, and may require prompt consideration.

Outside Toxins and the Effect They Have on the Liver

We have seen the need to eat nourishments that will help detox the liver, and how infrequent liver detoxification to flush poisons out of the framework is useful. In any case, how would we maintain a strategic distance from these poisons in any case? You may be acquainted with a panic that has turned into a web sensation over the harmful impact of a vehicle's cooling framework; there is a considerable amount of disinformation out there also. I won't go into it here, yet teaching yourself on every one of these issues will help you expel these bits of gossip.

In any case, it is evident that we all, and particularly those with persistent liver disease, ought to be wary against significant levels of natural poisons. We can have more noteworthy genuine feelings of serenity to lessen our introduction to toxins are:

1. Maintain a strategic distance from all tobacco smoke. This means more than just not smoking, you must also avoid second-hand smoke too. The vast majority comprehend the harm tobacco smoke can do to the heart and lungs. However, it likewise negatively affects the liver. The poisons in smoke lead to constant aggravation and scarring in the liver cells, prompting cancer and liver fibrosis.

2. Farthest point gas smolder presentation. Those vapors indeed are terrible for you. The liver will evacuate these poisons, yet on the off chance that severely strained, the liver may become overpowering. Much will rely upon the presentation's length and power, yet the more that can be stayed away from, the better. There are filling stations now that have fume recuperation frameworks to catch the exhaust. This incorporates maintaining a strategic distance from gas contacting your skin.

3. Comprehend that benzene-containing synthetic compounds are unsafe. You can smell them with solvents, artistry supplies, and paints. This is frequently because of benzene, a lethal synthetic that can add to an over-burden of liver danger. It used to be utilized as an added substance to gas yet has been diminished in on-going decades. For items that contain benzene be sure the region is all around ventilated.

4. Breathing in exhaust vapor can be dangerous. If you are sitting in rush hour gridlock; there might be little you can do to abstain from breathing these exhausts. One choice is to hold the windows down and change your vehicle's ventilation framework to re-course. At present, there will be some poisonous vapor in this air, yet positively not almost to the degree the outside fumes exhaust from sitting vehicles.

Chapter 8

FOOD AND HERBS

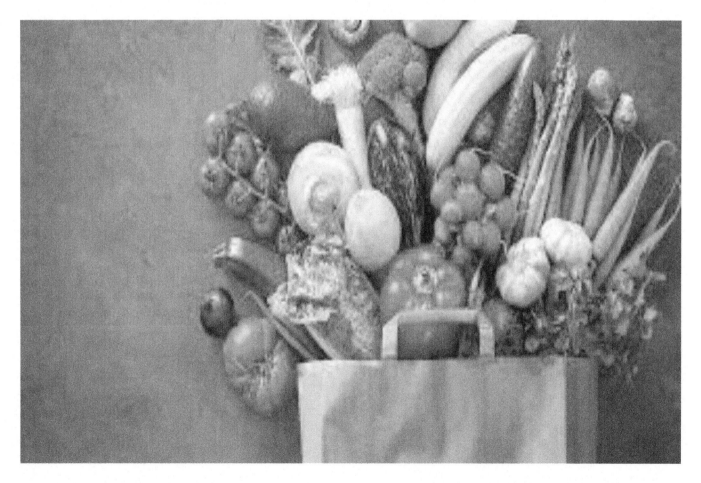

Natural and Unnatural Foods

Dr. Sebi breaks down foods into two groups: natural and unnatural. As soon as you hear these familiar terms, you might think you already know what Dr. Sebi is talking about. However, Dr. Sebi uses the terms "natural" and "unnatural" differently from what you might expect. When you think of "unnatural" foods, you are likely to think of fast food, processed food, and other unhealthy, human-made products. While these types of food are considered unnatural according to Dr. Sebi's diet, the category is much broader. Many foods that grow naturally, which most people would consider natural, are considered unnatural in Dr. Sebi's system due to them being high in acidity. Dr. Sebi explains that, while a plant such as burdock is "natural", other kinds of produce like aloe vera and peppermint are unnatural and too acidic for human consumption.

Dr. Sebi's Approved Food Items from Each Food Groups

Dr. Sebi Vegetable List

As for all his electric products, Dr. Sebi claimed that people could consume products other than GMOs. That involves fruits and vegetables rendered seedless or modified to produce more minerals and vitamins than naturally. Dr. Sebi's vegetable list is very broad and varied, with many choices for making multiple diverse meals. This list contains:

- Arame
- Amaranth
- Bell Pepper
- Avocado
- Cherry and Plum Tomato
- Chayote
- Cucumber
- Dulse
- Dandelion Greens
- Hijiki
- Garbanzo Beans
- Kale
- Izote flower and leaf
- Mushrooms except for Shitake
- Lettuce except for iceberg
- Nori
- Okra

- Nopales
- Olives
- Purslane Verdolaga
- Tomatillo
- Onions
- Sea Vegetables
- Squash
- Turnip Greens
- Wakame
- Watercress
- Zucchini
- Wild Arugula

Dr. Sebi Fruit List

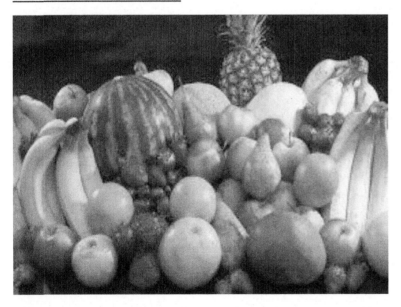

While the list of vegetables is lengthy, the list of fruits is very restricted, and certain varieties of fruits are not allowed for consumption when on a diet by Dr. Sebi. However, the selection of fruit is still providing a broad range of choices to diet followers. For example, on Dr. Sebi's food list, all kinds of berries are permitted besides cranberries, a fruit made by man. The list also includes:

- Bananas
- Berries
- Apples

- Currants
- Dates
- Figs
- Cantaloupe
- Cherries
- Grapes
- Limes
- Mango
- Prunes
- Raisins
- Soft Jelly Coconuts
- Melons
- Peaches
- Pears
- Plums
- Prickly Pear
- Sour soups
- Orange
- Papayas
- Tamarind

Dr. Sebi Food List Spices and Seasonings

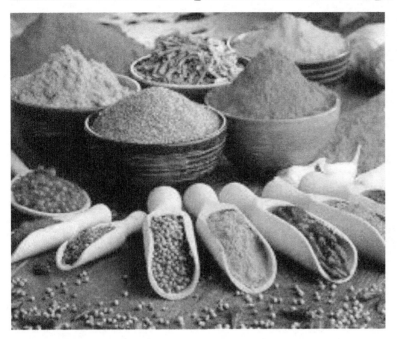

- Bay Leaf
- Cayenne
- Cloves
- Achiote
- Basil
- Dill
- Oregano
- Habanero
- Powdered Granulated Seaweed
- Onion Powder
- Tarragon
- Thyme
- Pure Sea Salt
- Sweet Basil
- Sage
- Savory

Alkaline Grains

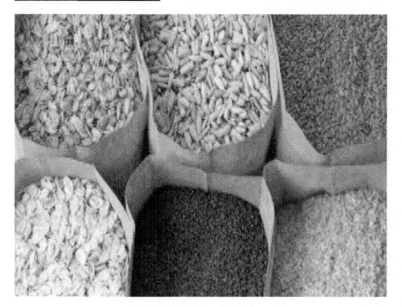

- Kamut
- Amaranth
- Fonio
- Quinoa
- Tef
- Rye
- Spelt
- Wild Rice

Alkaline Sugars and Sweeteners

- Coconut sugar
- 100% pure agave syrup from cactus
- Date sugar from dried dates

<u>Dr. Sebi Herbal Teas</u>

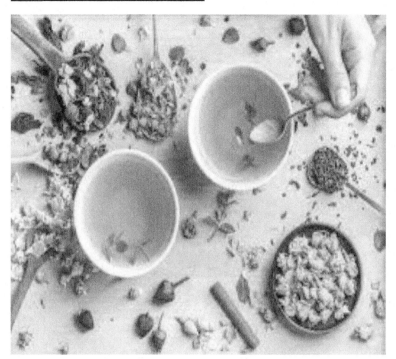

- Elderberry
- Ginger
- Red Raspberry
- Burdock
- Chamomile
- Fennel
- Tila

Nuts and Seeds

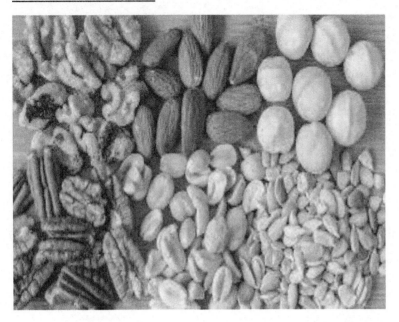

- Walnuts
- Brazil Nuts
- Hemp seeds
- Raw Sesame Seeds

Oils

- Olive Oil
- Coconut Oil
- Grapeseed Oil
- Sesame Oil
- Hempseed Oil
- Avocado Oil

Chapter 9

FOOD ASSOCIATION

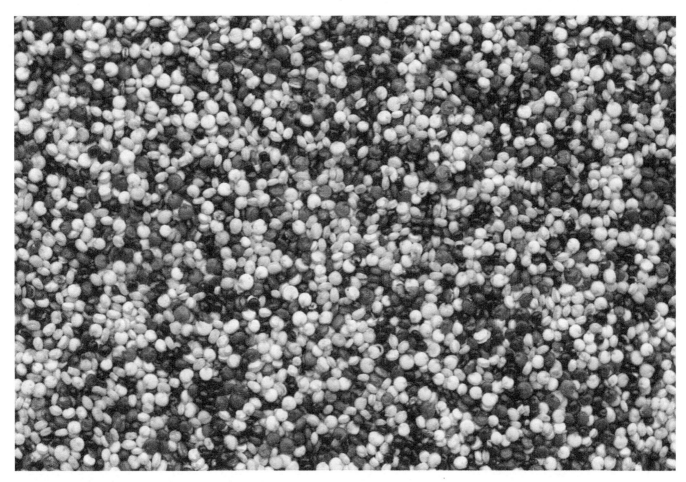

Dr. Sebi divides the foods into six main categories:

- Live
- Raw
- Dead

- Hybrid
- Genetically modified
- Drugs

For better health, you should have mostly live and raw foods. Such foods are alkaline and will heal your body from the damage done by acidic foods like meat, seafood, alcohol, sugar, processed items, and fried foods. Dr. Sebi also restricts all human-made, genetically modified, and hybrid foods. Seedless fruits, insect resistant, and weather-resistant crops also should be avoided, like corn, certain types of tomatoes, foods with added vitamins and minerals.

His diet plans recommend leafy greens, ripe fruits, non-starchy vegetables, and nuts. You can also have some grains like rye, quinoa, Kamut, but it will be better to minimize or eliminate other grains from your diet.

His dietary regime is specially designed to eliminate toxins, waste, and acidic elements from the body. By switching to such an alkaline, plant-based diet, you will lose weight and your health will be much better than now.

Dr. Sebi created this nutritional food guide or food list himself but with time many items have been added or removed and here you will find an updated list.

Can I Only Eat Foods from This List?

If you are committed and wish to try this diet plan, you will have to follow it strictly. Do not go astray from this list. In the beginning, you may feel it hard to stick to the list, but soon you will find that it is completely normal and you can do it.

It is hard; it is true, especially today's modern lifestyle where there are wrong foods everywhere. Sometimes, it becomes impossible to stick to a strict diet schedule. Therefore, you will have to be prepared mentally and emotionally and study and research hard to enhance your knowledge and skills.

Advice for Beginners

It doesn't matter if you are presently on this diet plan or not, as a beginner, it will be best for you to not get too involved with the approved food list for now. Otherwise, you will feel that you are left with only limited meal options for you.

It will be more important for you to gradually change your existing diet by replacing junk and other foods with more natural foods at the beginning stage. It will help you gradually.

Chapter 10

DR. SEBI'S NATURAL FOOD GUIDE TO END DIABETES

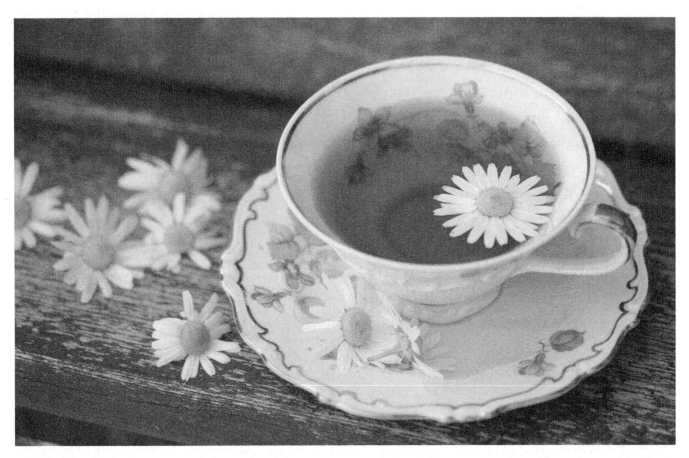

Although it is quite difficult to plan a diabetes food as it does not necessarily need to have a taste or to be boring, with just a little direction, a diet plan that is both nutritional and delicious can be conjured up.

Diet Planning

A dietetic plan should ensure that all the carbohydrates taken in each diet every day are well spread out not to engulf the body system. This is vital as it assists in making sure that the blood sugar levels are kept in control. Therefore, there is a requirement to stay on the pathway of what is being eaten.

The number of carbs eaten can also be controlled while making use of insulin and performing exercise. The majority of diabetic patients have to be worried about the sodium content of the foods they eat. It can play a negative part in the high blood pressure present in most diabetic patients.

Those with an extra medical condition of hypertension would be conscious of taking in sodium. For diabetic patients with high levels of lipids while taking in saturated fats, cholesterol, and trans-fat would be watched.

While trying to create a meal plan for a diabetic patient, some basic points should be noticed. These might add to ensuring that the calories taken in are kept to about 10% to 20% from a protein source.

Meats, which include beef and chicken, should be thought about over other options. About 25% to 30% of the calories should emerge from fats. However, foods that have saturated and trans fats should either be eaten in bits or shun. About 50% to 60% of calories should emerge from carbohydrates. Taking in plenty of oranges and green vegetables will help you sustain the balance, they may include broccoli or carrots. Taking in sweet potatoes or brown rice is preferable rather than regular potatoes and white rice because it is more advisable to eat as it serves as a nutritional benefit. This is a disease that builds because of the issue associated with the hormone insulin, which is produced by the pancreas. In cases where this process is interrupted due to irregularity, there is not enough control of the blood's glucose and the amount taken into the cell. However, a few of the medical and home remedies can be taken a look at to control this abnormality within the body.

Natural Sugar Control

Outlined below are a few recommendations of home remedies that should be taken a look at when you want to reduce the problems of diabetic patients:

- Taking alpha-lipoic acid helps manage the blood sugar level, and it is seen as one of the best multipurpose antioxidants.

- Taking 400mcg a day. Chromium picolinate helps insulin to keep the sugar levels in the body low. The Chromium picolinate keeps the blood sugar level when you take the right insulin.

- Taking garlic is another essential method of assisting the circulation and control of sugar levels. It comes in suitable capsules for easy and stress-free consumption.

- 500mg of L-glutamine and taurine each day will help bring down the sugar cravings and release the insulin the right way. It is useful for people who have problems managing their intake of sweet food items.

- Huckleberry is the best option for improving insulin production in the body when taken with the right prescription. It is a natural remedy that is recommended for consumption.

- A mixture of tea and kidney beans, navy beans, white beans, lima beans, and northern beans helps eliminate the pancreas' toxin.

There are more natural remedies that are used in managing blood sugar levels in diabetic patients. Meanwhile, the listed remedies should be consumed with either medical authorization or advice from some experts who have a deep understanding of the diabetic disease.

Type 2 diabetes affects over 30 million Americans – and the diabetes epidemic shows no sign of getting eradicated. When a patient has type 2 diabetes, it requires the sugar level to be controlled. When diet and exercise fail to control the blood sugar level, medications like metformin become an alternative. But with the breakthrough Dr. Sebi gave in his research for alternative medicines that help cure diabetes, we now have a huge list of herbal medicines that can not only control the blood sugar level but have the potential to cure it.

The research of these herbs has been proven to work in treating type 2 diabetes. According to Dr. Sebi, a combination of electric food is needed to keep the body's alkalinity at the level it needs to repel mucus.

Root Vegetables and Fruits for Diabetics

Because of the several health problems that can happen in a person with diabetes, it is necessary to be careful with the diet plan taken every day.

Fruits and Veggies

Any food consumption needs to be done with some level of sensitivity to make sure it is the best for the diabetics. Every diabetic patient needs to make sure they follow a balanced diet rich in minerals and vitamins. Also, the foods which have protein, fats, and carbs should be at an acceptable level.

Root vegetables and fruits have been taken as a huge source of minerals and vitamins and fiber which is vital in reducing the chances of heart attack and stroke. These root vegetables and fruits generally assist in making up for any side effects of the distressed blood sugar level. These side effects are expected to lead to heart attacks and blindness if not managed effectively by regulating minerals and vitamins obtained from the root vegetables and fruits.

It should be noticed that eating root vegetables and fruits is a mixture of other food items that are seen as the best for diabetic patient consumption rather than eating them without taking in snacks. It is so because when these root vegetables are eaten together with other foods, the chemical reactions will let all the vitamins and the minerals to be easily absorbed in the body system and this will lead to a controlled blood sugar level.

However, when taken in as a standalone item like snacks, the blood sugar levels are likely to be increased as the absorption levels will be twisted and lower than optimum. The most vital point to take notice of is to make sure that any food you eat should be done in a mixture that lets the absorption levels be the best for the patient with diabetics to take in.

Chapter 11

THE BENEFITS OF THE DIET

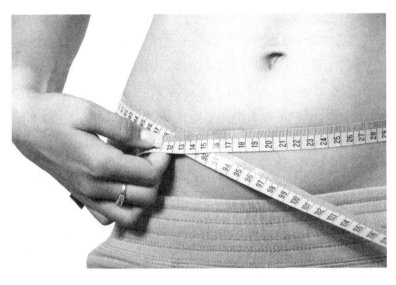

Dr. Sebi's diet offers a lot of benefits to the dieters. While the foods recommended from this diet are known to reduce inflammation, there are other benefits that you can reap from following the Dr. Sebi Diet.

Weight Loss

While this diet regimen is not for weight loss, it can help people who want to lose weight. Studies show that people who consume an unlimited whole plant-based diet experience significant weight loss compared to those who follow the Standard American Diet. How people lose weight with this diet relies on the high fiber and low-calorie foods encouraged to eat. Except for avocados, nuts, seeds, and oil, most foods encouraged by the Dr. Sebi Diet are low in calories. But even if you consume nuts and seeds, they are calorie-dense and rich in fiber and minerals.

Appetite Control

Although many people think that this diet is very restrictive in terms of the number of calories a particular person takes in, studies indicate that this diet can help with appetite control. The high fiber in your food can provide a high satiety level and make one feel full longer.

Altering the Microbiome

The stomach is the second brain. The enzymes and molecules released by the microbes in the gut affect not only your health but even your everyday mood. What you put into your body also affects the molecules that the microbes release into the bloodstream. The type of food that you also consume can also affect the kind of microbes in your stomach. For instance, studies show that consuming greasy, fatty, and processed foods can lead to the decline of good microorganisms and promote the growth of bad bacteria in the body.

Reduced Risk of Disease

While inflammation is one of the body's first lines of defense indicating infection and diseases, chronic low-dose inflammation can also be bad to the body. Chronic inflammation can result in many kinds of diseases such as diabetes, stroke, and even cancer. Thus, diets rich in fruits and vegetables are linked to reduced inflammation caused by oxidative stress. Studies that look into individuals consuming plant-based foods have a 31% lower chance of developing heart diseases and cancer than those who consume animal products.

The many restrictions of the Dr. Sebi Diet make it hard for some people to stick by it. Before you decide to give up because this diet demands a lot from you, below are helpful tips that you can follow to become successful.

- Research about Dr. Sebi's methodology: Following this diet has several rules that you need to know. Before you adopt this diet, you need to do due diligence by reading information.

- Download the nutritional guide: Make sure that you download the nutritional guide to serve as your guide when choosing ingredients to cook your Dr. Sebi Diet-approved meals. You can also use the nutritional guide to make your meal plans.

- Prepare your weekly meal plan: Making a weekly meal plan will organize your pantry and allow you to think of delicious meals that will keep you inspired and motivated to continue following the diet. Planning your weekly meal plan will also help you know how much food you need to buy or stock in your pantry.

- Plan your shopping trips: Planning your shopping trips is especially important when following the diet. Schedule your shopping trips especially if you need to buy your ingredients from different places. By organizing your shopping trips, you will be able to buy all the ingredients to create delicious meals for the week.

- Do fasting: The diet is all about allowing your body to detoxify. To help with this process, you can also do fasting to jumpstart the detoxification of your body.

- Find support: Find like-minded people to give you the morale boost that you need while following the program. Look for groups within your community or online who also follow the diet.

How to Follow the Diet

To follow Dr. Sebi's diet, you need to adhere to his rules present on his website strictly. Here is a list of his guidelines below:

1. Do not eat or drink any product or ingredient not mentioned in the approved list for the diet. It is not recommended and should never be consumed when following the diet.

2. You have to drink almost one gallon (or more than three liters) of water every day. It is recommended to drink spring water.

3. You have to take Dr. Sebi's mixtures or products one hour before consuming your medications.

4. You can take any of Dr. Sebi's mixtures/products together without any worry.

5. You need to follow the nutritional guidelines stringently and punctually take Dr. Sebi's mixtures/products daily.

6. You are not allowed to consume any animal-based food or hybrid products.

7. You are not allowed to consume alcohol or any kind of dairy product.

8. You are not allowed to consume wheat, only natural growing grains as listed in the nutritional guide

9. The grains mentioned in the nutritional guide can be available in different forms, like pasta and bread, in different health food stores. You can consume them.

10. Do not use fruits from cans; also, seedless fruits are not recommended for consumption.

11. You are not allowed to use a microwave to reheat your meals.

Chapter 12

DETOX WITH THE DR. SEBI DIET

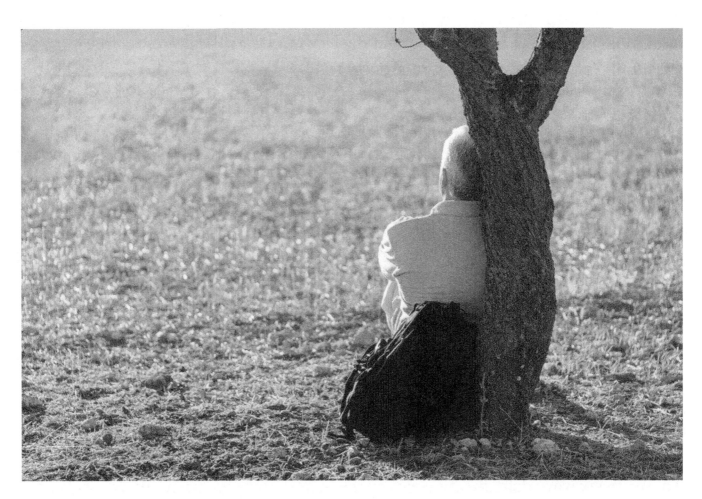

What is Detoxification?

From the first day of conception till death, we are exposed to various kinds of foreign chemicals daily. This has been greatly increased by modern living. These chemicals could be toxins from the environment, industrial properties and chemical waste, pesticides, medication, inorganic chemicals, heavy metals, etc. The chemicals may enter the body through the air we breathe or the food we ingest. These chemical composites are foreign because the normal biological system does not recognize them, and hence, they are known as xenobiotics.

The process by which the body is cleansed by getting rid of these xenobiotics is called detoxification. And yes, the body was designed to self-detoxify and excrete these xenobiotics through either sweating, urination, or excretion. And the principal organ responsible for cleaning the body is known as the liver. But because of the continuous exposure to these chemicals daily and stress, our body isn't always capable of carrying its natural function. This is because even the food required to support the body with necessary minerals and vitamins to aid it in carrying out its duties is now mostly refined. And as such, it leads to the reduction of original nutrients and, hence, less of the essential nutrients required to carry out the human system's detoxification process fully.

These chemicals do not cause problems immediately but over some time after accumulation. This is known as the ramification of toxic overload, and it differs from person to person. MCS, which is an abbreviation for multiple chemical sensitivity, is a possible effect of toxic presence. MSC is a situation where an individual experiences different symptoms because of exposure to different chemicals. These symptoms may include fatigue (which is the most common symptom), depression, headaches, illness, joint and muscle pain, mental confusion, irritability, flu-like symptoms, cardiovascular disorders, stuffy nose, etc. Although MSC is common when persons are exposed to chemicals from petroleum and coal-tar, it also develops after long-term consistent exposure and accumulation to some kinds of xenobiotics at home or in various workplaces. Toxic overload would most likely lead to inflammatory and rheumatoid arthritis and some neurological diseases such as Alzheimer

Types of Detox

There are six ways detoxification can be done, and these forms are named below:

- Physical detox
- Mental detox
- Emotional detox
- Energetic detox

- Surroundings detox
- Spiritual detox

Physical Detox

Usually, when the word "detox" is mentioned, this detox is what comes to mind. It is important to note that processed white flour, sugar, white rice, and harmful chemicals should be avoided when detoxing. Juice could be added to the regimen for physical detox; however, it is not necessary.

Mental Detox

A person's mind can be either one of two things; a tool that has massive power, or a threat that can bring destruction. This means that if a person's mind is unclean, that person's life can prove to be extremely difficult as a result. The fastest and surest way of detoxing the mind is through affirmation, mantra, and Hekau combined with meditation.

Emotional Detox

Human emotions are affected and influenced by factors such as food, social media, and the internet, music, and so on in the world today. The problem is that these factors bring about an excess of emotions that are unhealthy. The most effective method in cleansing human emotions is intelligence. Be that as it may, the brain of any human being is incapable of functioning from an emotional standpoint and an intellectual standpoint at the same time because these two are in separate parts of the brain. A state of calm, clarity, internal assessment (self-contemplation), and awareness will cleanse the emotional body. Emotional detox is capable of cleansing negative emotions, but this cannot be done directly; for example, traffic congestion is brought about by excess overcrowding of vehicles on the road. So, to clear this traffic jam, a path must be created that allows vehicles' free vehicular movement.

Simply put, detoxing the emotions is sort of like clearing up a road with traffic congestion. Once this is done, every form of thought that seems clogged up will then have a free flow. Later, those thoughts have to be brought to mind in ambiance where clarity is the mainstay because if that does not happen, they will be buried and become clogged up once more.

The following are some ways to bring an environment or atmosphere of intelligent clarity into existence:

1. Clean your space, let in sunlight, and expose it to fresh air.
2. Engage in spiritual practices or exercises that demand self-examination.
3. Using the Urban Zen's BRAKE tool (BRAKE = Breathe, Relax, Assess, Known, Engage).

Energetic Detox

In many traditional cultures, depression is defined as "Energy Down" – what this means is that it is seen as a lack of life force and resonance. As a result, a person's life force can either be boosted or cleansed although it is recommended that both are needed to remove certain things that could be responsible for the continuous drain in the life force.

Outlined below are the ten ways by which life energies can be cleansed and/or boosted:

1. Salt Baths (Cleanse).
2. Baking Soda (Cleanse).
3. Frankincense or Sage (Cleanse).
4. Pyramid of Light – Guided Meditation by URBN Zen.
5. Bee pollen and Yohimbe (Boost).
6. Laughter (Boost).
7. Herbs for energy such as Rhodiola, Ashwagandha, Ginseng, Basil, and so on.
8. Dancing or movement (Boost).
9. Music or sound healing (Boost and Cleanse).

Surroundings Detox

Often, detoxing the surroundings or environments we find ourselves in is usually neglected, be that as it may, it is also very crucial, and it brings about more flying results. Surroundings or environmental detox can generate an ambiance for the other forms of detox to thrive.

The following are some of the crucial things to think about when you go about detoxing your environment:

1. Toxic people.

2. Harmful chemicals.
3. Radiation.
4. Conversations that may come off as toxic – in essence, observing mute days.
5. Music.
6. Television.
7. Electronic devices.
8. The internet and social media.
9. Properly cleaned and organized home.
10. Keeping living and common spaces such as your home, car, work, or desk, purified.

Spiritual Detox

Spiritual detox is also referred to as ablution – originally, a practice where a priest washes his hands or items that are regarded as sacred – and it is the most powerful of the other kind of fast and permeates through the others. This means that, when the different forms of detox are combined with ablutions, the effect will be amplified to a great extent. However, with detox, ablutions are a spiritual exercise in which the mind, the body, and the spirit are purified with certain substances considered as having divine powers which are the elements and chemicals. It is recommended that every day is started and ended with ablutions to ensure the home remains clean. Be that as it may, ablutions are only the first feature to consider when spiritual detox is concerned.

The following are some of the features of a spiritual detox:

1. Ablutions.
2. Fasting.
3. Praying.
4. Spiritual work at the proper time and place (that is, zemzems).
5. Mantra, Hekau, or chanting.
6. Meditation on pure or spiritual principles as well as thoughts.
7. Submitting or restraining of the senses or pleasure.
8. Chemical cleansing (this is usually done with water charged with divine force).

Benefits of Detox

There are an innumerable number of benefits that can be derived from using detox, and the benefits that are received are dependent on the particular detox used. The range of benefits obtained from discus is the purification of impurities physically, mentally, emotionally, energetically, proximally, and even spiritually.

Outlined below are some of the confirmed results that have been brought about from following through with either one or all of the six detoxes:

- Improvement in energy level.
- Loss of weight.
- Reduction of stress.
- Emotional and mental clarity.
- Clear skin.
- Alleviated constipation.
- An end to headaches.
- Reduction in pain.
- Restfulness and relaxation.
- Control of cravings
- An end to corruption.
- Promotion of a healthy environment.
- An end to food addiction.
- Thwarting of long-lasting diseases.
- Enhancement of immune function.
- Improvement in the quality of life.
- Readjustment of bodily systems.

Detoxing gets rid of excess accumulation of blood or other fluids in the system and promotes optimum health.

Chapter 13

THE DIFFERENCE BETWEEN PHLEGM AND MUCUS

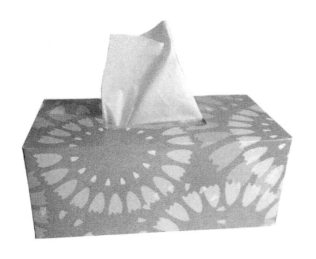

Phlegm Carries Disease

Phlegm is very difficult to expel from the body. The presence of phlegm in the body is an indication that there is a disease lurking around somewhere in the body. When phlegm is excreted in the body, mucus accompanies it as well as bacteria. This is the more reason why phlegm is more problematic to the body.

Mucus and Disease

It is ideal to know the concept of diseases, the environments where it thrives, and the causes. With this knowledge handy, it will be difficult for us to fall sick. This is the key to staying away from diseases and illnesses that your doctor will never tell you about. There won't be the need for a healer as getting sick will be a rare occurrence when we know these things.

Mucus Is the Cause of Every Disease

Diseases are found in the body when you have ingested an uncomplimentary substance into our body. This substance will conflict with our genetic structure, which will eventually lead to us getting sick and weak. Almost everyone usually gets sick due to excess mucus in the body. The cause of most diseases is the presence of excessive mucus in the body.

When mucus accumulates excessively in the body, the mucus membrane breaks down, and cells get covered by the excess mucus. In essence, the mucus membrane is to protect the body from the invasion of aerobic bacteria.

Mucus and Phlegm Cause Disease

When our diet is made up of acidic food, the mucus membrane breaks down, and the already secreted mucus gets into the bloodstream. When this happens, the other groups of cells that belong to the organs get deprived of oxygen. If the mucus travels to your nostrils, it is referred to as sinusitis, when it flows to a bronchial tube, it is called bronchitis, and when it enters the lungs, it is called pneumonia. If mucus manages to get into your eyes, there will be a problem with vision.

- Prostatitis – when mucus gets into your prostate gland
- Endometriosis – when mucus gets into a woman's uterus (this can lead to yeast infection and vaginal discharge).

When you have the symptoms of any of these diseases, excessive mucus production caused by an inadequate diet is the underlying cause.

Phlegm After Eating

Humans experience phlegm every other time. When you cough out phlegm after eating, it is as a result of you consuming acidic food. Now you understand that the excessive acidic food you consume causes you coughing out phlegm. One of the significant factors contributing to the excessive production of phlegm in the body is the consumption of processed foods. The body does not notice these foods, and it in turn results in a conflict. If you find yourself producing a lot of phlegm via cough after eating a particular type of food, you need to stay away from such food. The production of excess phlegm due to the consumption of a particular type of food indicates that such food is unhealthy. The secretion of excessive phlegm will deprive the body of oxygen and other parts of your internal organs.

Symptoms of Constant Mucus in the Throat

Acidic foods do not complement the biological structure of the human body. The body's reaction to this is to produce more mucus every time you eat acidic foods. Excess mucus in the longs will extend to the throat. This situation will lead you to cough out phlegm after every meal you take.

A temporary solution to this condition is to gargle saltwater, but a diet change is needed to stop the body from producing excess mucus. If you refuse to change your diet to eliminate the excessive production of phlegm, there will be more of it to cough out every time you consume acidic food. Every organ of the body that hosts this excessive mucus will experience one disease or the other.

Common Remedies to Clear Mucus:

Have a 2-7 day juice fast to enable your body to scrub and flush out the bodily fluid/mucus joined by a blended diet of foods grown from the ground suggested by Dr. Sebi.

Boiled a quart of water, include half tsp. of lobelia, and let it steep. When it is tepid, strain it, and drink as much as could reasonably be expected. Stick your finger down your throat so you can regurgitate to free your stomach from mucus and bodily fluid.

Before this, take a hot shower quickly make the water cold and run it on your body. Hit the hay, at that point have somebody give you a hot fomentation to your chest and spine and finish it with a cold one - this is to diminish blockage.

Remember, changing your eating regimen is the most significant thing you can do to help your body deliver an abundance of mucus and bodily fluid.

Chapter 14

DETOXING AND REVITALIZING YOUR BODY

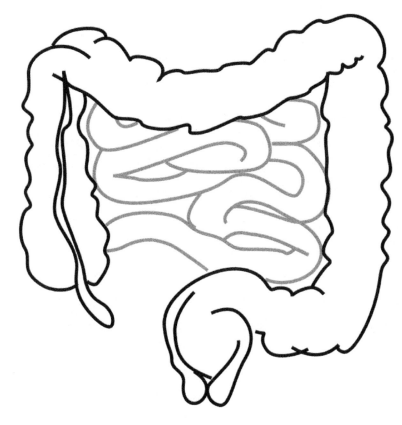

The human body is always working to remove toxins and unwanted substances from several organs in the body. As time goes on, the human body gets weakened due to the consumption of unhealthy foods, alcohol, drugs, caffeine, stress, and we can also add to the list. These environmental toxins are present everywhere due to the increase in industrial waste.

Despite the conscious effort, you might take in maintaining a healthy diet or lifestyle; several external factors always put our body's system in an unhealthy state. Our body is then required to remove such factors that may prevent us from enjoying optimal health. When our essential and functional organs are made to work due to toxins' presence, over time, they tend to get tired and become less efficient, which may lead to illness.

Setting out time to cleanse the body system and help reduce the stress these organs undergo will go a long way to prevent any further disease. This approach has immediate and visible effects such as increased energy level, clearer skin, faster and better digestion, etc. This now begs the question, what is detoxification?

Detoxification, often called detox, is the elimination of harmful, poisonous, or toxic substances from the human body, through medical or physical means which is carried out mainly by the liver. It can be referred to as the time frame of withdrawal which enables the organism to get back to homeostasis after a long duration of consuming additives. In medicine, detoxification can be facilitated by the removal of poisonous ingestion and the use of antidotes. Techniques such as dialysis and chelation therapy can also be used, but only in a few cases.

Where Do Toxins Come From?

In times past, we grew our food naturally making use of natural means such as fertilizers, composite manure, and pest control. That era is fading speedily as we now rely heavily on refined and packaged foods with lots of preservatives, factory-farmed meat, fish, and milk.

The major problem is that this modern era of farming makes use of pesticides, synthetic fertilizers, and enhanced hormones. Also, foods that are genetically modified (GMO) permits the use of many herbicides and pesticides. Genetically modified foods and their well-spread products have increased the levels of toxins we consume.

These toxins, when combined with air-borne pollutants such as carbon monoxide from the exhaust pipes of cars, pollutants from manufacturing companies, and Agricultural wastes and pollutants disposed of in our water bodies, can prove catastrophic. Our drinking water also contains traces of chemicals such as chlorine used in treating the drinking water.

Types of Detoxification

Alcohol Detoxification: Alcohol detoxification is a process whereby your body system that contains too much alcohol is cleansed and brought back to its normal state. Alcohol addiction results in the devaluation of GABA neurotransmitter receptors, and a hasty removal from long term alcohol addiction without proper medical administration, can lead to severe and fatal health problems. Treatment of alcoholism is not alcohol detox, but after detoxification, other treatments should be undergone to scrap the addiction caused by alcohol usage.

Drug Detoxification: Drug detoxification is used by clinicians to bring down withdrawal symptoms while it helps an addicted individual adjust to living without the use of drugs. Drug detoxification stands for early steps within long term treatment but does not aim to treat addiction. Detoxification can be accomplished without using drugs or may use medications as a part of treatment. Drug detoxification and treatment often occur in community programs that last some months, and it also takes place in residence locations instead of a medical center. Drug detoxification changes reliance on the placement of treatment, but some of the detox centers provide treatment to avert the symptoms of physical withdrawal from alcohol and other drugs, these additions include therapy and counseling during detox to help with the effect of withdrawal.

The moment you realize an imbalance in your health; then that is the right moment to reclaim it. But it is always difficult when the kickbacks gotten from long gluttony weighs heavy on you, in this case, a detox can be beneficial as an adequate remedy. People experience lethargy due to lack of sleep, being too low on energy, and not being active in everyday activities. Definitely, you will want to rejuvenate your whole system and carry out some detoxification processes on your body and mind.

According to Mary McGuire of the American Yogini in Rosenberg, New York's American Yogini "Just like the spring and winter cleaning you do for your home, it's great to do the same with your body and detoxify twice a year as the seasons change."

For you to detoxify yourself, it means you have some reasonable level of discipline and dedication. According to past detoxers, they testify on how it enhanced their energy, and increased their mental clarity, and even caused their skin to glow. If you are new to detoxing, the best results come to those who go on a retreat for a few days and experience a lifestyle completely different from their everyday edible toxins. You are advised to consume foods such as grains, fish, fiber, and forgo meat and instead concentrate on fresh, organic fruits and vegetable juice, and this will be a lot simpler to maintain when you are far from home.

Just a three-to five-day retreat brings back good energy, stress-free sleep, and general good feeling, and some people get to lose 5-7 lbs. within a week and up to 20 lbs. within two weeks. After the first three days of tasking discipline, people experience hunger pangs, cravings, and nausea due to the disappearance of low blood sugar.

Is Your Body in Need of a Detox?

Below are some signs to look out for:

- You get tired quickly due to stress.
- You feel constant headaches and a reduction in mental clarity.
- You sometimes experience skin breakouts and blemishes, not bright, and have a poor complexion.
- You easily get colds, bugs, flu, and some viruses, and most times you are on medication.
- You sometimes experience trouble, like an uncomfortable digestion process.
- You frequently eat less-healthy foods such as fried foods, iced meat, dairy, refined foods, refined sugar, etc.
- You often take coffee, drugs, cigarettes, alcohol, etc.
- You frequently encounter environmental toxins such as cigarette smoke, carbon emissions, pesticides, herbicides, and chemicals used at home.
- You feel heavy due to excess body weight.
- You continuously experience depression, due to unstable emotions and you lack the required energy to carry on, also you have low enthusiasm for life generally.
- You sometimes experience bad breath and body odor no matter how often you brush your teeth or bathe.

Chapter 15

UNDERSTANDING HOW YOUR BODY DETOXIFIES ITSELF

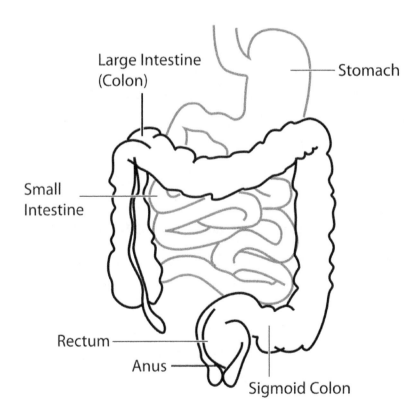

The marvels of the body do not cease to amaze me. When you truly consider what your system is capable of accomplishing, I wager you are astounded also. Among the most notable things that your body would be to treat the influx of toxins.

From the mouth to your own skin into your kidneys -- and also lots of areas and components in between -- your own body is installed to help you prevent and cleansing yourself. I believe that it's essential to grasp all of the methods by which your system copes with poisons so you can play a significant part in helping out it and strengthening its detox procedures. That is what I concentrate on during this chapter. Have a spin over the upcoming few pages to learn what's happening within the human own body to help keep your well-being from an environment that continues to become more hazardous with every passing season.

Your Mouth: Chewin' It Up

All digestion begins in the mouth area. Food and fluids enter the human body through your mouth and a few really important things happen there. Powerful and healthful digestion expects that your mouth is performing its own work, and your own body's capacity to cure itself can be significantly helped if you make a bid to permit your mouth to perform its work. Remember when your mother told you to slow down and chew your food? This was great advice. Whenever your teeth grind your meals into smaller pieces, your meals are much better able to experience the numerous measures. Chewing your food nicely enables your gut and intestines to break the food down and extract its own nourishment using a greater level of efficacy. The end result is a healthy you across the board, plus it is a hell of a lot easier for your body to fight toxic risks if it is healthy. But that is only one detoxification worth that chewing the food provides.

If you chew thoroughly rather than consuming larger pieces of meals, you also make it a lot easier for the acid from your gut to break the food down. Stomach acid is still a great toxin fighter, and you also wish to observe that your body is just taking advantage of its own powers, so make sure you chew your food completely before consuming it.

Besides chewing gum, the mouth adds a component that is essential for digestion: spit. This superb fluid does all kinds of things:

Binds and Lubricates

The mucus at saliva makes the meals you consume quite glossy, and it contrasts the meals together in a soupy mix that slips down your stomach without damaging the liner of the significant tubing that runs from the mouth into your stomach.

Allows You to Flavor Dry Food

Without spit, it might be almost impossible to flavor food that is dry. In the event that you were eating something with poisons which may be tasted -- foods spoiled by damaging, poisonous germs, for example -- you likely would not even understand it.

Lactic Acid

If you consume highly acidic foods, there is always a possibility that the acidity may damage your own mouth (such as your own teeth) and stomach. Saliva includes sodium bicarbonate, and it can be a compound that reduces acidity. Sure, your gut is extremely acidic, and following your food there it becomes completely saturated in acidity. However, your gut lining is made to manage acids in a manner your mouth and nostrils only cannot.

The Digestion of Starches

Saliva releases a compound that starts to break down starches into fundamental sugars. That is a fantastic thing as your body can not do at all with starches, although it has to possess sugars (for electricity) to endure.

Kills Germs

This can be a large one. Saliva includes a chemical known as lysozyme that may kill bacteria in your meals and also the germs that attempt to increase inside your mouth and in your own teeth. You also understand that a few kinds of bacteria may be just as poisonous as the worst chemical compounds, therefore it is of the utmost significance that you are not bringing elevated levels of germs in your body once you place food into your mouth. (A side note: Compounds cause bad breath. Healthy levels of saliva kill more germs, thereby assisting you to prevent bad breath.)

Simplifies Dental Hygiene

Saliva constantly melts away plaque debris, which can be a significant reason for bad oral hygiene. This information really surprises a few folks, but you should not drink fluids with your meals. Doing this simply is not great for digestion. In the event you have to wash off your food with fluids, you are not chewing enough, and you are not letting the food become penetrated by and coated in spit. You are also diluting the acid from your gut, and it can be a significant part of the practice of killing poisonous germs before it passes their own intestines. Many pharmaceutical medications decrease saliva and can lead to a very dry mouth if you've got this issue, speak with your physician. My advice would be to wait for a few hours after a meal before drinking fluids. Following that, you are able to drink all of the water you desire.

Your Stomach: Breaking' It Down

In case your body needed a garbage can, it might become your gut. Whenever your sinuses utilize mucus to trap particles of dust, mildew, viruses, and germs, where does this mucus find yourself? On your gut. Whenever your mouth happens in foods and fluids which could contain harmful, poisonous germs, where does this stuff end up? On your gut. If the tubes resulting in your lungs snare foreign substances from the atmosphere you breathe until they return to a sensitive lung tissue, where can they ship these substances? That is right up -- your windpipe, in your stomach, then down to your tummy.

Your tummy is tough, hard, and prepared to undertake just about anything that you put into it. Would you blame it on perusing each once in a while?

Giving It to the Germs

The secret to the gut's wonderful capability to deal with virtually all your body yells its stomach acid. This is not some weak acid such as the type on your lemon juice. If your stomach acidity has been sitting on your table rather than on your gut, you would soon be on the marketplace for a new table. It is even powerful enough to consume metal away, which means that you may imagine the effect it will on most poisonous substances that end up on your gut once you accidentally eat, drink, or inhale it. Your stomach acid breaks down various kinds of harmful toxins, and also the wellness of your gut is a significant element in maintaining the human body as toxin-free as you can.

Stomach acid can destroy almost whatever's living as it reaches your stomach. Because you can imagine, this capacity has significant benefits for the immune system. It is a great deal easier for your body to just kill things off such as dangerous germs, mildew, and parasites on your gut than to take care of the ramifications of these creatures endangering your immune system.

Interfering with Your Gut's Workout

When stomach acid is more powerful and current in healthy quantities, it can be exceedingly tough for potentially dangerous household things to pass through the gut and input your intestines. But lots of people nowadays take drugs -- both prescription and over the counter -- for both abdominal pain or indigestion, and thus reducing the quantity and potency of acidity in the gut. These medications can help relieve stomach discomfort, but they also make it a good deal simpler for dwelling threats to living on your own body and finally offer your immune system matches.

If you are experiencing frequent tummy pain or indigestion, then be certain you and your physician consider several potential causes before you begin taking medicine that interrupts the acidity from your stomach. The pain may be brought about by a range of different items, and you also do not wish to undermine the acid from your stomach if you don't have to.

If one of my patients encounters a burning sensation in her gut or signs of acid reflux, I test the degree of acidity in her gut. I really don't hope to find very significant levels of acidity; in reality, ordinarily (and particularly with elderly patients) the challenge is a deficiency of stomach acid. Difficult to believe? Here is how it works.

When it is working properly, your gut will not let food put in your intestines before the food is partially digested. If you do not have sufficient acid in your stomach, the food is not digested well enough along with your belly and hangs onto it rather than sending it on later on. Shortly your stomach starts to contract to the food that is delayed in a bid to attempt and combine it together with the tiny quantities of acid found. When it's five hours after you have eaten a meal and then you are lying down with a tummy full of food, and your belly starts contracting, you are certain to get pain or acid in your stomach.

This chain of events is common in elderly patients. A greater proportion of elderly folks are taking powerful acid-reducing medicine than before. If this were the ideal solution, the reason would need to be the elderly folks are generating higher quantities of stronger stomach acid because they age. This would indicate that the cells from the gut are functioning better in their own attempt to create more acid. But let us be fair: virtually anything works much better as we get old. In such scenarios, it might well be the acid-reducing medications are a more demanding therapy. If you believe that could be creating your gut troubles worse by taking medications that reduce down in your stomach acid, then make sure you bring the query with your physician prior to taking any actions. The most important thing is that almost all acid reflux can be caused by low acidity -- not large acid. The great news if you are acid reflux is the fact that the issue is relatively simple to fix. It's possible to choose an old medication known as sucralfate that does not lower acidity levels but can help cover some raw stains on your gut lining which may cause you pain. (The most frequent brand name for sucralfate is Carafate.) You're able to take advantage of this medication together with betaine HCL, which can help acidify your belly to the ideal amounts when you are ingesting a meal. That mixture will fix stomach pain issues in a lot of men and women. But please do not take these measures until consulting with your physician.

Processing Protein

As well as killing off harmful compounds, the acidity in your stomach works to break down proteins to amino acids, and your body needs to have to be able to survive and flourish.

With no gut's processing of protein to amino acids, then you would not have the ability to digest and consume those materials into your blood, and you would have difficulty staying healthy for long. Maintaining up healthy levels of acidity in the stomach is vital here. In the event you utilize acid-reducing medications unnecessarily, then you might be placing your nourishment in danger.

Your Intestines: The Centre of Detox Action

It is difficult for many people to think, however, your big and tiny intestines are a joint 30 ft. in length. That is the length of a soccer field's end zone! Along with the absolute dimensions of your intestines compared to that which they do if it comes to sorting out fluids and consuming the ideal nutrients in the human body. They are excellent body components, and a lot of the detoxification effort set forth from the entire body takes areas throughout that 30-foot span.

Your intestines hold thousands of small folds known as villi. They include a large amount of surface area into the intestines -- thus far, in reality, they make the entire region of your intestines that is readily available for absorption about the exact same dimensions as a tennis court! Villi are accountable for absorbing distinct substances from the partly digested food that moves. Whatever they consume is passed to your blood and consequently made accessible for the body to utilize. They are not likely to consume toxins, naturally (whatever your body does not need must pass through with your feces) but a few toxins possess a chemical structure which permits them to get beyond the villi and in your blood.

Generally, your intestines do a good job of consuming the nutrients that you want and ridding the toxins which may harm you. But if you do not get enough of the prior and you are earning much too much of this latter, then it may cause some significant problems on your own intestines. I should not need to inform you just how important it's to keep up the well-being of a 30-foot manhood that's responsible for the absorption of nearly all of your body's nourishment.

Bringing the Barrier

Once you consider it, the walls of the intestines are the one thing between your own body's cells along with your feces. It is an amazing and quite protective obstacle, and it is nearly magical in its ability to allow the fantastic things to pass in your body while retaining the awful things going through together with your own waste.

Along with supplying a superbly energetic physical obstacle, the intestines also incorporate a great deal of important components of your own body's biological barrier against infection: the immune system. It is a little-known actuality that about 80% of your body's immune system can be found in your gut. Even the GALT (gut-associated connective tissue), situated largely towards the end of the small intestine, is that the last barrier which divides the interior of the human body from the feces, which at the point usually comprises dangerous items such as toxins, bacteria, yeast, and mold, and parasites.

Taking in a lot of toxins by your diet plan may endanger the health of your intestines, such as the GALT. That scenario makes it tough to keep up the integrity of the physical barrier and also the resistant barrier, and illness is frequently the outcome. If you wish to maintain your intestinal hurdles working as they need to, do everything you could to remove toxins in the daily diet.

Regular Flora

Your intestines play some vital purposes, but in addition, they behave as a boarding home for the majority of the beneficial bacteria inhabiting your physique. The ordinary, healthy bacterial flora in your intestines plays an essential role in digestion and breaking several distinct sorts of food your body is not able to break back by itself.

The standard flora in your intestines also gives you different support. When existing in healthy quantities, the beneficial bacteria consume space and nutrient sources which may otherwise be employed by damaging, poisonous organisms such as yeast, bacteria, and parasites.

Removing the Clutter

The chemical reactions and processes which happen in your intestines if nutrients have been consumed and toxins are closed out are equally as complicated and refined as anything you would find in the most technologically innovative chemical firm. In addition to this, your intestines possess an extremely complex manner of transferring your partly digested foods and feces through at a suitable speed, so that every one of the procedures can happen in the ideal quantity of time. This function can help to keep poisons going through and finally from your entire body. In case your intestines proceed things too quickly, diarrhea (which may have a devastating impact on your nourishment and hydration degrees) is frequently the outcome. If your intestines move too slowly, constipation may happen. Whenever your feces spend longer on your intestines as it needs to, you are simply giving the toxins from your feces longer to hang about and get accidentally absorbed into your machine.

There are lots of autoimmune diseases that traditional doctors typically treat with medication that helps control the symptoms but does not do anything to tackle the reason for the issue. A number of these disorders, such as Crohn's disease, ulcerative colitis, and irritable bowel syndrome, which may be significantly exacerbated by the existence of a lot of toxins in the diet plan, and detox diets frequently go a very long way toward supplying relief.

Chapter 16

DR. SEBI'S FOOD NUTRITION PHILOSOPHY

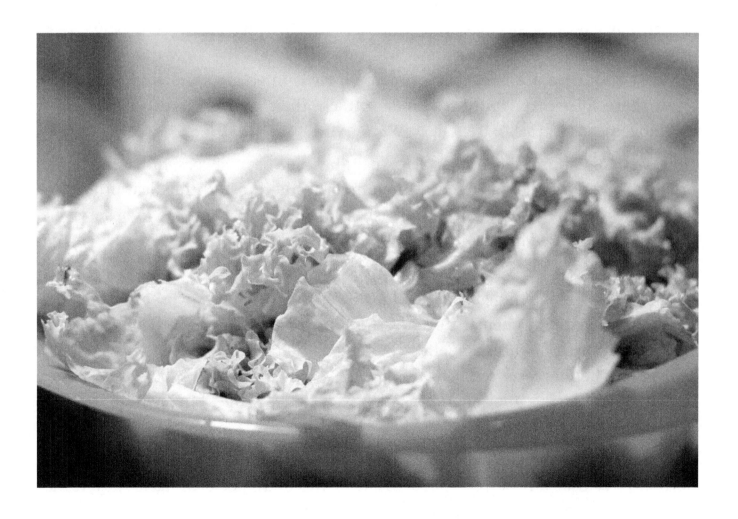

Life Energy

A big part of Dr. Sebi's philosophy is the great distinction between life and death. Dr. Sebi has a saying, that "One must consume life – not death – in order to maintain and sustain oneself." It is acidic foods that are considered unnatural and are associated with the death of the body. Damage to the mucus membrane, excess mucus spreading throughout the body, stagnant toxins flooding the organs, and the eventual disease and illness that results, all stem from the root of unnatural foods (or acidic foods). Alkaline foods are viewed as being alive and contributing to life energy. They restore balance to the body, and the organs that are undernourished due to excess mucus are healed up and restored.

Basics of the Food Nutrition Philosophy

Dr. Sebi's diet has as its core in maintaining and improving health or wellness (which earned him the alias the 'wellness guru') by returning the body to its original alkaline state. Western medical research holds the view that diseases in the host result from a bacterium, fungal or virus infection. And that in order to treat these diseases, you first must attack their causes, and then employ carcinogenic chemicals to treat it.

However, this approach for over 400 years has not been successful, as it has not provided to be a sustainable cure. In contrast to the Western medical procedure, the wellness guru believes illness and disease are a result of and can only survive in mucus and an acidic environment (that is, a compromise in the mucus membrane).

For example, excess mucus in the lungs would lead to the disease known as pneumonia, in the bronchial tube it leads to bronchitis, etc. So, using inorganic chemicals to treat diseases is ineffective and self-defeating because they contain an acid-base. Therefore, in treating these diseases, it is more beneficial to use natural herbal remedies since they alone can effectively detoxify the body by returning it to its original alkaline state.

Although, toxins which eventually build up the acidic level of the body are normally released in the body as a result of the body performing its day to day functions (these are known as endogenous). He also believes that among other things like our environment and lifestyle, the kinds of food we eat have a crucial role to play in either maintaining, increasing, or even reducing the level of acid or alkaline in the body.

The reason for this is because they could end up producing exogenous toxic chemicals (toxins from the outside) in the body. Dr. Sebi divided these foods into six primary groups which are raw, live, dead, drugs, genetically enhanced or modified, and hybrids.

Dr. Sebi went further to divide the particle contents of food into two categories; positively charged ions (for example, chloride, phosphate, and sulfate) and negatively charged anions (for example, potassium and calcium). When foods containing these particles are broken down or digested, they form either alkaline or acids in the body, respectively.

However, ingesting and digesting this food might not immediately result in any trouble. Still, over a period of continuous ingestion and digestion, it leads to the accumulation of toxic acidic waste which will invariably lead to acidosis (a very high acidic environment). In this type of environment, health begins to deteriorate, and illness and disease would continue to thrive.

So, according to this nutrition philosophy, our body needs to always be in an alkaline environment for it to remain healthy and carry out its functions effectively. Dr. Sebi's whole diet goal is to regulate the alkaline level of the body using the food we ingest as the principal tool and some herbal supplements which his company produces.

So, among Dr. Sebi's six food categories listed above, only raw and live foods are permitted to be taken. The reason for this is that he considers them to be "electric foods." He further restricted approved foods in these two categories to only plants which include vegetables, fruits with seed, grains, etc.

Dr. Sebi's diet excludes the consumption of animals and all their associated products entirely. Hence, this diet could be referred to as 'an alkaline vegan diet'.

What is a Vegan Diet?

A vegan diet or veganism is a more complex and stricter form of a vegetarian diet. While a vegetarian diet prohibits the consumption of animals such as poultry, fish, and meat, a vegan diet goes further to prohibit all animal products such as dairy, eggs, etc. A vegan diet is a strict plant-based diet! There are several types of vegan diets which may include:

Raw food diet: These are foods based on raw vegetables, seeds, fruits, or even botanical foods cooked below the temperature of 118 degrees Fahrenheit or 48 degrees Celsius.

All-food vegan diet: These are foods based on all foods that are plant-based such as grains, nuts, legumes, vegetables, fruits, etc.

Starch solution: Based on a plant food that is low in fat and rich in carbs. It has as its primary focus cooked starchy foods such as rice, potatoes, and corn instead of fruits.

Raw till 4 p.m.: This diet is deficient in fat and prohibits the eating of raw food after 4 p.m. it, however, allows cooked plant-based food for dinner.

80/10/10: This diet, like the starch solution, also limits plant food that's rich in fat (for example, avocados, nuts, etc.). This vegan diet focuses mainly on soft vegetables and raw fruit, and it is also known as a fruitarian diet or raw food vegan diet.

Junk vegan diet: This vegan diet allows the consumption of cheese, fries, fake meats, vegan desserts, and all other vegan food that are heavily processed. Beginners to the vegan diet would easily find this vegan diet appealing.

Thrive diet: This diet allows the consumption of whole plant-based foods raw or at most a little heated up at a very low temperature. Like 80/10/10, it is also a raw-food vegan diet.

It would be correct to say that Dr. Sebi's diet (that is, all foods on his recommended and approved food list) are foods in the vegan diet. But not all foods in the vegan diet are on Dr. Sebi's approved food list. The reason for this is because while veganism focuses on all plant-based foods, Dr. Sebi's diet focuses on specific plant-based foods that are alkaline.

Simply put, food that helps regulate the body's pH to its original alkaline state by producing positively charged ions. Some of these foods include ripe fruits with seeds, quinoa, Kamut, non-starchy vegetables, rye, avocado, bananas, cauliflower, grapes, lemon, chamomile, ginger, walnut, etc. A detailed list would be given in the next chapter. However, there are some principles to adhere to when following an alkaline vegan diet that we should consider:

Principles of Eating a Vegan Alkaline Diet

Ensure to ingest (eat) a lot of high quality fresh whole foods: when following an alkaline diet, the idea is to eat fresh whole foods grown without genetic modifiers (GMO) and in several varieties. So, sticking with an alkaline vegan diet would focus on eating a variety of plant-based foods which include fresh fruits; squeezed or whole, fresh vegetables; raw (whole or juiced), and lightly cooked, slightly toasted nuts and seeds. In these forms, we could ensure that the foods retain their active and essential ingredients. Note, for full health benefits, a wide variety of these foods is required. The reason for this is simple; repeated consumption of a particular food does not only limit your necessary nutritional types but also disrupts digestion. This would also ensure the digestive system is given the room to develop fully, by trying out different varieties of food and flavors.

Ensure you consume 60-80% alkaline foods: the 60-80% range would ensure you get the maximum benefits of an alkaline diet whether you choose to follow the diet in order to remain in good health or to restore good health and then maintain it. In the first case, at least 60% of the foods containing a positive charge or also known as alkaline-forming foods should be eaten. While in the second instance, at least 80% of these foods should be eaten. So, it is recommended that you find alkaline-forming foods you enjoy in order to meet this requirement.

Avoid eating food that is not friendly with your immune system: for this reason, it is highly recommended that you carry out an LRA test so that you know what you are allergic to. This would help you plan out an all plant alkaline diet that your immune system won't be reactive to.

Follow the recommended healthy nutrient ratio: this is a critical ratio that will ensure you get the necessary amounts of nutrients in the right proportions. This principle would balance your intake of plant-based carbohydrates, protein, and fats. The recommended ratio is as follows below:

Complex carbohydrates should make up about 60 – 70% of your overall food intake. These carbs could either be gotten from grains, legumes; to include lentils and peas, vegetables, herbs, or spices.

For protein, about 50 to 60g per day is recommended. And this should amount to about 15 – 20% of your calorie intake. These whole plant sources include seeds, mushrooms, sprouts, legumes, etc. However, during pregnancy, your protein requirement would increase.

The recommended ratio for healthy fats is about 15 -20% of your entire calorie intake. However, we must be particular about getting omega-3 essential fats for enhancing and improving our body's energy production abilities, tissue repair, and also the production of proteins (for example, enzymes). Omega-3 crucial fats from plants include fresh seed and nuts, organic cold-pressed oils (such as olive oil, walnut, avocado, safflower, peanut, sesame, grape seed, black currant, *etc.*). Omega-3 supplements could be used, but you must ensure that the ingredients or components are from whole plants.

Plant-based proteins from a single plant when compared to animal proteins, lack essential amino acids. So, to fully get the required amino acids, it is highly recommended that plant-based food be paired. The following lists are examples of food pairing that would complete your required protein:

- Beans and brown rice or corn.
- Grains with plant-based milk.
- Grains with legumes, seeds, or nuts.
- Chopped walnuts and brown rice.

Consume food and drinks that are pro-biotic: These foods and drinks are known to promote life, which is the aim of an all alkaline vegan diet. These life-promoting foods could either be fermented or cultured. These foods and beverages are the major sources of probiotics that facilitate healthy gastrointestinal tracts.

These tracts in turn house numerous pro-biotic bacteria which play a very important role in balancing our immune system and body in general. When these bacteria are depleted, maybe as a result of illness, stress, poor dieting, or even antibiotics, harmful pathogens are given room to develop freely. Examples of probiotic foods and drinks include yogurt (nondairy), kombucha (a fermented tea), sauerkraut (a fermented cabbage), kefir (a fermented milk), olives, fermented soya beans (known as tempeh), pickles, freeze-dried microalgae, etc.

Take a lot of fiber and water: There is a general belief that staying disease-free requires the consumption of about 40 to 100 grams of fiber from whole plant food daily. This is very correct and for this reason, we recommend that you consume at least 40 grams of fiber per day. The reason for this is because fibers contain roughage, which aids the digestion and excretions processes.

It not only cuts down transit time (that is, the period between the time of ingestion of food and the waste products from the food are ejected from the body), it also adds to one's stool to make it bulky. A balanced intake of fibers facilitates the regular, easy, and convenient elimination of toxic which will invariably prevent the body from accumulating and reabsorbing toxic waste. Note, 12 to 18 hours is the range of a healthy transit time.

While water is very important to healthy living, it not only regulates the body's temperature but also aids the easy removal of waste products from the body, especially when on a fiber diet. It is recommended to take about eight cups of water a day. Drinking water about 30 minutes before and meals improve the body's process of digestion.

Consume different varieties and combine healthy foods: Just like we discussed in principle 4, following a whole plant alkaline diet would require a healthy combination of foods in order for you not only to get the necessary nutrients, but also to get them in the required proportions. In fact, because of the shortage in necessary nutrients, a single plant-based food can provide, one cannot really talk about following a healthy vegan diet without talking about food combinations.

Apart from the above facts, it also aids the digestion process which invariably affects the body's health in general. Food combinations also reduce wear and tear on the system of digestion, which is associated with repeated consumption of the same food. Note, when combining foods, you should be on the lookout for simple and compactable foods.

Rules for Following Dr. Sebi's Diet

When following Dr. Sebi's diet, it is compulsory to obtain Dr. Sebi's herbal cell supplements and use them religiously in order to receive maximum results of the diet. There are also specific rules to adhere to when following his diet plan and these rules are as follows:

- The only plant-based foods you must consume are foods listed on Dr. Sebi's approved list of foods.

- You must drink a gallon of natural spring water daily.
- When taking any Dr. Sebi's supplements, they should be taken over an hour before the application of any medication.
- Avoid the consumption of animals and all their products, as well as all hybrid and genetically modified foods.
- Avoid the intake of alcohol.
- Avoid the consumption of grains that are not naturally grown and found on Dr. Sebi's approved list. And also, completely stay away from consuming wheat.
- The only fruits allowed are fruits containing seeds. And also, avoid eating canned foods.
- On no account should your food be microwaved. The reason for this is because microwaves kill your food.

Chapter 17

MYTHS AND FACTS ABOUT ALKALINE

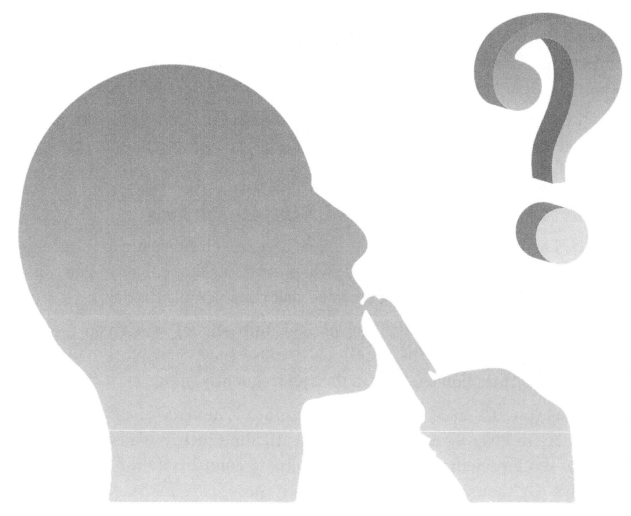

After 50, your body doesn't process nourishment how it did when you were more youthful. Your digestion eases back down, and you're bound to lose bulk and see changes in your weight.

Subsequently, it requires somewhat more thought and exertion to ensure you get enough alkaline and remain a healthy weight, says Alkaline dietitian Nancy Farrell. "I'm not into telling others that they ought to maintain a strategic distance from explicit nourishments," says Farrell, a representative for the Academy of Alkaline diet and Alkaline dietetics.

Conditions identified with undesirable Alkaline diets - like diabetes, weight, respiratory failures, and strokes - will, in general, happen all the more regularly as we age. So, individuals more than 50 need to watch their calories more intently and eat less nourishment with included sugar or a ton of big fats, similar to the ones in spread or shortening.

Specialists state that men more than 50 who are tolerably dynamic ought to get somewhere in the range of 2,200 and 2,400 calories per day. For ladies, that number is around 1,800 calories. Monitoring that is simpler since the administration began expecting cafés to post carbohydrate contents on their menus.

That is the sort of information that proves to be useful when you're attempting to remain sound more than 50. There are still a few misguided judgments out there that specialists are trying to clear up.

Myth: Since My Digestion is Slower, I Have to Eat Less

Not really, Farrell says. As you age, it might be more enthusiastic for your body to take in and use nutrients and minerals like nutrient B12, calcium, zinc, or iron. What's more, a few prescriptions can make that considerably harder.

Also, numerous grown-ups don't get enough nutrient D, which you require for bone and muscle quality. This usually is because they need more dairy in their Alkaline diets, or they don't get out in the sun frequently.

That implies you may need to eat a more significant number of certain things and less of others to ensure you get the correct Alkaline diet. For instance, you may need to eat more protein and get more exercise to compensate for the loss of bulk, Farrell says. Or then again, you may require more leafy foods, Dawson-Hughes says.

Myth: Supplements Are Good for You, So More Is Better

Since your body makes some harder memories getting supplements from nourishment as you age, numerous more seasoned individuals take calcium or nutrient D enhancements to help keep their bones reliable.

Myth: I'm Not Hungry at Present, So It's OK to Skip Dinner

There are advantages to keeping an ordinary calendar. "Your body is a campfire," Farrell says. "In case you have a blaze, you're going to toss another bit of wood to keep that fire consuming. That keeps the digestion fully operational. ... The caution is you must toss the correct quality and a pleasant quantity, not overcompensating either."

Fact: It's Past the Point Where It Is Possible to Change My Propensities.

"I see patients who have significant ailments and incessant sickness expresses that are deteriorating, and they are looking to slow the procedure," Farrell says. "They wish they would have been progressively genuine about wellbeing and Alkaline diet in their more youthful years."

Be that as it may, while it might be harder to change a few propensities, the more you've had them, "it is rarely past the point of no return or too soon to deal with conduct changes in any period of life."

What's more, skirt the arrangement supper at your nearby drive-through, Farrell says. Sugary beverages or treats, nourishments made with margarine or shortening, or nourishments produced using refined grains, similar to white bread or pasta, pack more calories with a less Alkaline diet.

"Things that don't include any Alkaline diet worth yet include calories will be fulfilling and cause you to feel full, and afterward, you will get inadequate in supplements that are significant," Dawson-Hughes says.

Fact: The Alkaline Diet is Everything

The high Alkaline diet isn't always about what you bring home from the store. At times, the test is finding a workable pace in any case.

Loads of things can influence how well you eat as you age. Losing teeth may make it harder to surrender certain nourishments; for instance, or your faculties of taste and smell can be changed as you get more established, Farrell says.

"Warm chocolate chip treats new out of the broiler don't have a similar impact any longer," she says. What's more, a few seniors have physical issues that make it harder to get around, or they don't have transportation. Money related issues, sadness, or seclusion are increasingly regular as individuals age, as well.

Chapter 18

THE PLANT-BASED ALKALINE DIET

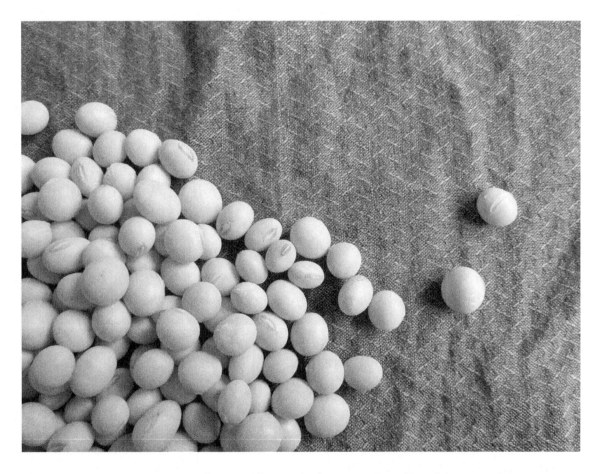

The Health Benefits of the Plant-Based Alkaline Diet

If you are a vegetarian, vegan, or aiming to move in this direction, the alkaline diet is ideal. While all dietary plans can be built on a strong foundation of vegetables and fruits, a plant-based diet is one of the best options for adhering to this way of eating. Not all vegan or plant-based diets are alkaline; a lot of foods that are free of animal products can be processed and contain acidic ingredients, though once digested, many "acidic" fruits and vegetables become alkaline. One of the most beneficial, nutrient-rich foods for an alkaline diet is soy. Soybeans (edamame beans) are a great snack on their own, as is tofu, tempeh, miso, and other soy-based foods. When choosing soy products, look for organic, natural options, and avoid preservatives as much as possible.

Why Choose a Plant-Based Diet?

There are many reasons for moving to a plant-based diet, from reducing meat in your diet overall, to implementing one or two "meat-free days" each week. If your current diet is very meat-heavy, this will take some major adjustment, so it is best to not make the switch from red meats to full veganism overnight. Veganism or vegetarianism works best when whole, natural foods are chosen instead of packaged or processed options. A lot of marketing is involved in promoting meat-free packaged snacks and condiments, though many of these may contain sugars, high amounts of sodium, artificial color, additives, and other ingredients that are unhealthy.

There is a lot of research to support a plant-based diet, and the high amount of alkaline in many fruits and vegetables means a good fit with the alkaline-based diet:

The emphasis is on whole, natural foods, which simplifies the process of shopping and selecting foods for your diet. This also makes meal preparation and planning much easier, as your focus will be on vegetarian-based eating, without meat as an option, and little or no dairy.

- A plant-based diet can help with weight loss, as vegetables and fruits are digested and used much more quickly than meat and dairy products. There are also fewer calories contained in vegetarian meals, even where the actual portion size is the same or similar to a meal, including meat.

- Meeting your goal weight is a great achievement, and maintaining weight is another task. This can be done much more effectively with plant-based eating, as there are not only restrictions on meat and dairy consumption, but on processed foods, which sometimes contain meat by-products (gelatin) and a high amount of preservatives and artificial flavors.

- Soy is a major staple of a plant-based diet. The amount of calcium, protein, iron, and nutrients in soy products is comparable to meat, and with a fraction of the calories and fat. Soy is also relatively inexpensive and easy to find in most grocery stores. Tofu, tempeh, and edamame beans are popular ways to enjoy soy in almost any type of meal.

- Enjoying a plant-based diet can reduce or eliminate food sensitivities to dairy and meat products, as these are no longer a part of the diet. Other food allergies or sensitivities may be less of a factor, once a more pH balance is established in your body, as digestion becomes easier and health improves overall.

- The health benefits of a plant-based diet, especially vegan, where all meat by-products and dairy foods are eliminated entirely are numerous. From improving heart health and cardiovascular function to preventing cancer, type 2 diabetes, and many other conditions. Prevention is a big factor in why choosing a plant-based diet, as many conditions and diseases can be avoided in the first place.

The Benefit of Soy in an Alkaline Diet

When it comes to soy, there are a lot of studies and findings that result in positive outcomes and benefits of eating soy on the dangers of increasing estrogen and the impact of this on your health. Overall, soy is a healthy option for any diet, especially for plant-based vegan diets that avoid all meat products. For people with allergies to soy and soy-based products, some alternatives can be used to adhere to a vegan meal plan successfully. For most people, soy is a good option with the following advantages:

1. High in protein. Soy can provide just as much, if not more, protein in your diet than meat. In combination with a balanced diet that includes fresh vegetables and fruits, your body will receive more than the required daily protein.

2. Low in cholesterol: Plant-based foods are low in cholesterol, saturated, and trans fats, which makes them a good choice for good cardiovascular function and a way to prevent heart disease.

3. High in fiber. Soy, like all vegetables and fruits, is very high in fiber. Not only will you meet your daily protein, calcium, and iron requirements by switching to soy from meat, but you'll also receive a good dose of fiber with each serving, which increases metabolism and keeps weight at a healthy, manageable level.

4. Vitamin B12 and other nutrients considered only available in meat and meat-related products are also found in some soy products. Fermented soy, such as miso and tempeh, contains a sufficient amount of B12 to meet dietary requirements.

5. Vitamin D is often an ingredient in dairy milk, due to being fortified, though this can also be found in various soy products as well. While only a small amount of this vitamin is required, it's important that it's a part of your diet.

6. Soy products come in many forms, textures, and flavors. Soft tofu varieties, for example, can be used to create puddings, cakes, and smoothies. Firm tofu and tempeh can be marinated and fried, baked, or sautéed with any combination of vegetables and ingredients. Soymilk is a great alternative to dairy and can be used with cereals, in smoothies, milkshakes, and as a refreshing beverage.

7. Easy to digest. While some people have reported bloating and mild issues with digesting soy, in general, it's easy food for the body to digest and break down for nutrients.

Alternatives to Soy for a Plant-Based Diet

If soy-based foods are not an option for your plant-based diet, there are many alternatives to choose from. These foods contain high amounts of protein, calcium, and iron, which are found in meats and dairy products:

Coconut-Cultured Yogurt

Similar to dairy yogurt, vegan, coconut-based yogurt is made by cultivating bacterial culture from coconut to make a product with the same texture, nutrients, and a similar flavor to dairy yogurt.

Vegan Cheese

Most varieties of vegan cheese are soy-based, though a growing number of plant-based cheeses are made from vegetables and vegetable oils. The benefits of vegan cheese include a similar taste and texture to regular, dairy cheese. Vegetable-based cheese, as opposed to soy-based products, tends to melt easier, which makes this variety a preferred option for vegan grilled cheese and Mac-and-cheese dishes.

Almond, Cashew, and Coconut Milk

There are many non-dairy milk alternatives available at nearly every grocery store and local restaurant. Almond milk is becoming nearly as popular as soymilk, as well as other nut-based kinds of milk, including cashew milk. Some varieties include a combination of almond and coconut milk, or cashew and almond, for a pleasant, nut-like taste that works well in recipes, smoothies, and with cereal. More people are ditching dairy milk and cream for non-dairy options for their coffee and tea as well. Other alternatives include hemp and rice milk.

Nut Butters

Peanut, almond, and other nut kinds of butter are an excellent source of protein and energy. Just one or two spoons of these butters will provide a good boost of nutrients before a workout or an active day.

Other Soy Alternatives

Nuts and seeds can be added to stir fry dishes and salads, instead of tofu and other soy foods to boost the protein and calcium content. Olive oil and coconut oil are both good alternatives for baking and cooking vegetarian dishes. Both oils have a neutral flavor that works well with any combination of ingredients.

Alkaline Fruits

Fruits are an excellent source of vitamins, fiber, and energy, with natural sugars that can easily replace the need for sweet snacks and processed foods. When we shop for fruits, we tend to choose from a small circle or group of fruits that we are familiar with and comfortable with. The variety of limitations on what fruit we buy can depend on what's in season, how much of a budget we have to work with, and our cravings. Bananas, apples, oranges, and berries tend to be most popular, and for a good reason: they are delicious and easy to eat. Apples are best during autumn when they are in peak season and are available in many varieties that vary in texture, taste, and appearance. During summer months, it's the perfect time to enjoy fresh fruits, such as berries, bananas, and melons.

If you buy local, fresh fruits become less available during winter or colder seasons. Frozen fruits are another option to consider. They are just as healthy and more convenient, as they last longer and can be used at any time. Canned foods, even vegetables or fruits should be avoided, as they contain extra sodium and sugar, along with other additives.

Which Fruits Are High in Alkaline?

All fruits have a significant amount of alkaline, which makes them all good choices for an alkaline diet. The amounts vary depending on which fruit, where alkaline is either low, moderate, or high. Some fruits that contain acidic properties will convert to alkaline once digested, like tomatoes and citrus fruits, while others contain a high amount of alkaline before consumption:

1. Blackberries, strawberries, and raspberries. Berries are a great choice in an alkaline diet, due to their high amount of vitamin C and antioxidants.

2. Nectarines, like peaches, are high in alkaline and make a great snack on their own, or in a fruit salad.

3. Watermelons are not only high in alkaline but also contain a good amount of potassium and fiber. They are an excellent choice for a snack and especially refreshing during the summer season when they are more readily available.

4. Apples have more of an amount of alkaline that's more moderate to high, though they contribute a lot of nutrients that make them a preferred snack any time of the year. They can be enjoyed raw, stewed, or baked for a variety of dishes. Apples are also naturally sweet, which makes them ideal for desserts.

5. Bananas are high in potassium, fiber, and pack a lot of energy into just one serving. In fact, one banana can provide up to 90 minutes of energy: an easy and quick snack before a workout, hike, or going cycling.

6. Cherries, similar to berries, are high in alkaline and fiber. They also promote regularity and a healthy metabolism.

Are there any fruits to avoid? With an alkaline diet, virtually all fruits are good options, which makes the diet an easy process to follow.

Chapter 19

TIPS FOR SUCCESSFULLY FOLLOWING THE ALKALINE DIET

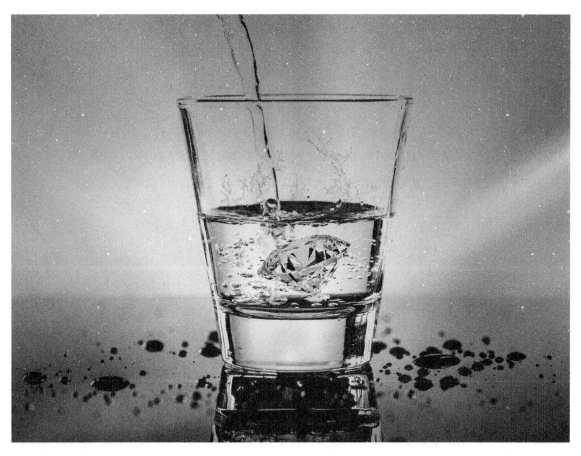

Often, stretching for the additional mile, you get to the areas you had only dreamed about. Going well on an alkaline diet will be the battle that ultimately contributes to a balanced lifestyle. An alkaline diet is an assumption that certain products, such as berries, vegetables, roots, and legumes, leave an alkaline residue or ash behind in the body. The body is strengthened by the key ingredients of rock, such as calcium, magnesium, titanium, zinc, and copper. The avoidance of asthma, malnutrition, exhaustion, and even cancer is an alkaline diet. Conscious about doing something like that? Here are ten strategies to adopt the alkaline diet effectively.

Drink Water

Water is probably our body's most important (after oxygen) resource. Hydration in the body is very important as the water content determines the body's chemistry. Drink between 8-10 glasses of water to keep the body well hydrated (filtered to cleaned).

Avoid Acidic Drinks Like Tea, Coffee, and Soda

Our body also attempts to regulate acid and alkaline content. There is no need to blink in carbonated drinks as the body refuses carbon dioxide as waste!

Breathe

Oxygen is the explanation that our body works, and if you provide the body with adequate oxygen, it should perform better. Sit back and enjoy two to five minutes of slow breaths. Nothing is easier than you can perform Yoga.

Avoid Food with Preservatives and Food Colors

Our body has not been programmed to absorb such substances, and the body then absorbs them or retains them as fat, and they do not damage the liver. Chemicals create acids, such that the body neutralizes them either by generating cholesterols or blanching iron from the RBCs (leading to anemia) or by extracting calcium from bones (osteoporosis).

Avoid Artificial Sweeteners

These sweeteners, which tend to be high in low fat, are potentially detrimental to the body. In addition, Saccharin, a primary ingredient in sweeteners, triggers cancer. Keep away from these things, therefore. Go for less healthy food, still a decent one.

Exercise

The alkaline and the acidic element will also be matched. This is not just a question of consuming alkaline milk. A little acid (because of muscles) often regulates natural bodywork.

Satiate Your Urges for a Snack by Eating Vegetables or Soaked Nuts

Whenever we are thirsty, we still consume a little fast food. Establish a tradition of consuming fresh vegetables or almonds, even walnuts.

Eat the Right Mix of Food

The fats and proteins of carbohydrates need a specific atmosphere when digested. And don't eat it all at once. Evaluate the nutritional composition and balance it accurately to create the best combination of all the nutrients you consume.

Use Green Powders as Substitutes for Food

This tends to improve the alkaline quality of the body.

Sleep Well and Remain Calm and Composed, Even When Under Stress

Seek to escape the pain. Our mind regulates the digestive system and only when in a relaxed, focused condition can you realize it functions properly. Relax, then, and remain safe!

Chapter 20

TIPS TO MAXIMIZE WEIGHT LOSS WITH EASE THROUGH THE DR. SEBI DIET

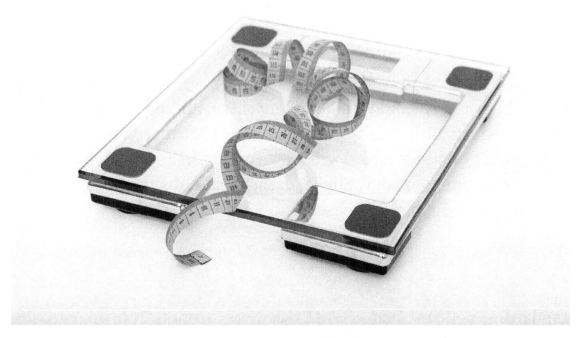

The Dr. Sebi diet advances eating entire, natural, plant-based nourishment. It might help weight loss on the off chance that you don't typically eat like this. Nonetheless, it intensely depends on taking the maker's costly enhancements, is exceptionally prohibitive, does not have certain supplements, and mistakenly vows to change your body to an alkaline state. In case you're hoping to pursue a more plant-based eating design, numerous healthy diets are progressively adaptable and practical.

Imagine a scenario in which you thought about a weight loss program that would assist you with getting in shape and feel more youthful. OK, attempt it? The alkaline diet and way of life have been around for more than 60 years, yet numerous individuals aren't acquainted with its regular, protected, and demonstrated weight loss properties!

The alkaline diet isn't a contrivance or a prevailing fashion. It's a healthy and straightforward approach to appreciate new degrees of health. It is right to say that you are getting a charge out of a thin and attractive body today? Assuming this is the case, you're in the minority.

Unfortunately, more than 65 percent of Americans are either overweight or hefty. In case you're overweight, you presumably experience indications of ill health like weakness, expanding, sore joints, and a large group of different signs of unexpected frailty. More terrible yet, you most likely want to abandon regularly getting a charge out of the body you need and merit. Maybe you've been informed that you're merely getting more established, yet that necessarily isn't reality. Try not to get tied up with that falsehood. Different societies have healthy, lean seniors who appreciate excellent health into their nineties!

Indeed, your body is a splendidly planned machine, and on the off chance that you have any side effects of ill health, this is a sure sign that your body's science is excessively acidic. Your side effects are only a cry for help. This is because the body doesn't merely separate one day. Slightly, your health disintegrates gradually after some time, at last falling into 'dis-ease.'

How Does Your Body React to The Hybrid Foods You Eat Now?

The Standard American Diet (S.A.D.) centers around refined carbohydrates, sugars, liquor, meats, and dairy. These nourishments are largely exceptionally acid-shaping. In the interim, in spite of supplications from the nourishing specialists, we don't eat enough of the alkalizing nourishments, for example, crisp organic products, veggies, nuts, and vegetables. To put it plainly, our S.A.D. way of life disturbs the universal acid-alkaline parity our bodies need. This condition causes stoutness, low-level throbbing painfulness, colds, and influenza, and inevitably disease sets in. We've lost our direction. This is the place an alkaline diet can help reestablish our health.

I'm sure you're acquainted with the term pH, which alludes to the degree of acidity or alkalinity contained in something. Alkalinity is estimated on a scale. You can take a necessary and reasonable test at home to see where your alkalinity level falls, just as to screen it routinely.

Medical analysts and researchers have known for in any event 70 years this lesser-known fact. Your body requires a specific pH level, or sensitive parity of your body's acid-alkaline levels - for ideal health and imperativeness.

We'll utilize two instances of how acid and alkalinity assume a job in your body.

We, as a whole, realize that our stomach has acid in it. Alongside proteins, this acid is fundamental for breaking nourishment into essential components that can be consumed by the stomach related tract. Consider the possibility that we didn't have any acid in our stomachs. We would die from lack of healthy sustenance right away because the body couldn't use an entire bit of meat or a whole bit of anything, so far as that is concerned!

Different pieces of our body require various degrees of acidity or alkalinity. For instance, your blood requires a somewhat more alkaline level than your stomach acids. Consider the possibility that your blood was excessively acidic. It would eat through your veins and conduits, causing a substantial inward drain!

While these models exhibit that the different parts or frameworks in the body need distinctive pH levels, we don't have to stress over that. We are essential to acidic, generally speaking, period. In case you're keen on getting familiar with pH, you can discover massive amounts of data on the web by basically looking through the term.

At the point when your body is too acidic over quite a while, it prompts numerous diseases like stoutness, joint pain, bone thickness loss, hypertension, coronary illness, and stroke. The rundown is unending because the body essentially surrenders the fight for imperativeness and goes into endurance mode as long as it can.

CONCLUSION

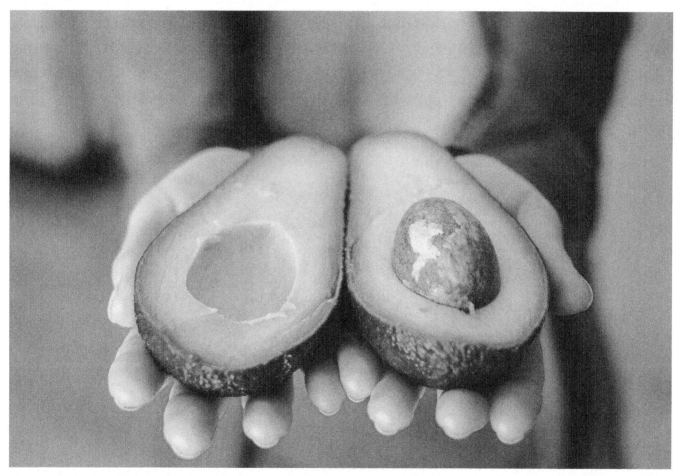

This diet approved by Alfredo Bowman, also known as Alfredo Bowman, allows certain food items that are 100% vegan and are not processed or modified. Dr. Sebi is not a professional and does not hold any degree but he claims himself to be a self-taught herbalist. Following this diet can help prevent diseases such as heart diseases, diabetes, kidney disorder, or liver diseases. This diet can also be used to reduce weight s. For quite some years, Dr. Sebi's diet has grown in popularity among the younger generation. This new trend is rising due to the poor healthy lifestyle of the current generation in terms of what they consume. So many fast foods are available to them, foods that contain harmful minerals that can cause a long-term problem like cancer. So, it is not a surprise that people are becoming more interested in natural means of flushing their system. Thus, the demand for Dr. Sebi's Alkaline Diet.

Detoxification and cleansing have several health benefits even if they have a few disadvantages. Some of the advantages are that it keeps you healthy and physically fit, boosts immunity, and improves the focus of the person. Other than that, there are also natural methods of detoxification such as dry brushing, cupping, souping, exercising, etc. By adopting this diet, one can have several health benefits that are shinier hair, healthy and clear skin, improved immunity, and overall optimal health. Herbs and Food Recipe provides the individual with a variety and versatility that will help to follow the diet approved by Dr. Sebi. There are a lot of combinations for the approved items that can be achieved and enjoyed.

Book 2

DOCTOR SEBI:

The Real 7 Days Healing Journey with a Balanced Alkaline Plant-Based Diet. 200 Easy and Tasty Recipes, Approved Food List, Detox Smoothies to Lose Weight and Boost Your Health.

Lauren Hill

INTRODUCTION

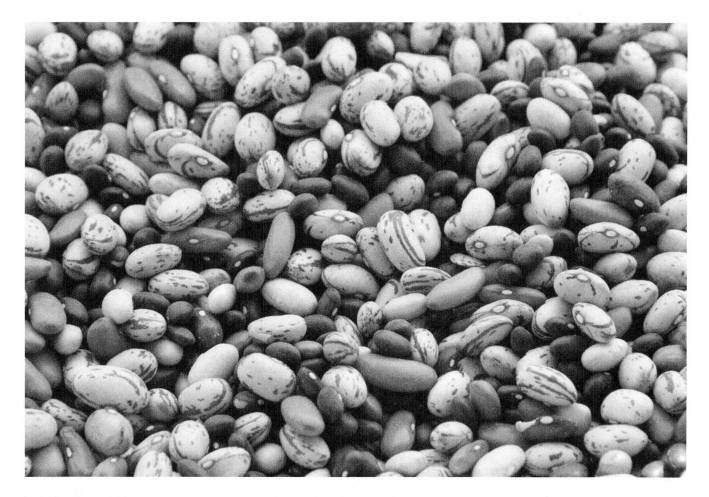

The Alkaline Diet and Intracellular Cleansing

The Alkaline Diet is a way of eating that balances your pH levels by choosing the right foods, mostly alkaline based, to maintain good health. Becoming familiar with the right types of food items to include in your diet is as simple as learning whether each item on your grocery list is alkaline or acidic.

Before your next trip to the supermarket, review the list of items or write down the foods you usually include on a typical shopping trip. For example, your list may contain the following items:

- Milk (2L)
- Bread
- Yogurt
- Apples (1 bag)
- Butter
- Ground beef (2 lbs.)
- Breakfast sausage
- Potatoes (1 bag)
- Eggs (1 dozen)
- Spinach (frozen)
- Case of pop/soda (12 cans)
- Tomatoes
- Mayonnaise
- Granola bars (1 box)
- Garlic

In total, there are fifteen items on this grocery list. How many of them are acidic versus alkaline? The results may be surprising:

Acidic: milk, bread, yogurt, butter, ground beef, breakfast sausage, eggs, pop/soda, mayonnaise, granola bars

Alkaline: apples, potatoes, spinach, tomatoes, garlic

Two-thirds of these items are acidic, while the remaining is alkaline. It is important to note that all the alkaline foods on this list are vegetables and fruits. In general, nearly all fruits and vegetables are alkaline-based, which makes a plant-based diet a good foundation to build an alkaline diet. The key is a balance, even with acidic foods as part of your regular diet, by increasing the alkaline content significantly over time. This will have a major improvement in your health in many ways.

Below is an idea of how your shopping list might look if you choose to follow Dr. Sebi's diet.

Fruit

Add any of the following Dr. Sebi-approved fruits to your shopping list:

- Bananas
- Apples
- Currants
- Berries
- Cantaloupe
- Dates
- Figs
- Tamarind
- Papayas
- Oranges
- Pears
- Plums
- Melons
- Peaches
- Cherries
- Grapes
- Limes
- Mangoes
- Raisins
- Prunes

Grains

Add any of the following Dr. Sebi-approved grains to your shopping list:

- Wild rice
- Kamut
- Amaranth
- Spelt
- Rye
- Quinoa
- Tef

- Fonio

Vegetables

Add any of the following Dr. Sebi-approved vegetables to your shopping list

- Bell peppers
- Amaranth
- Avocados
- Arame
- Dandelion greens
- Nori
- Lettuce (excluding iceberg)
- Mushrooms
- Garbanzo beans
- Kale
- Chayote
- Onions
- Tomatillo
- Olives
- Okra
- Squash
- Wild arugula
- Zucchini
- Wakame
- Watercress
- Turnip greens

Chapter 1

EXCESS MUCUS IN THE BODY

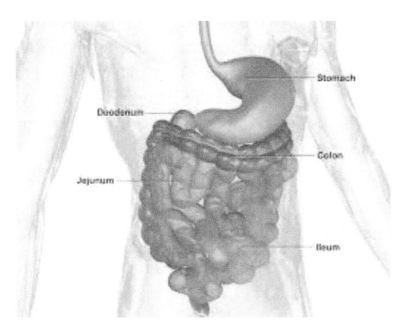

Mucus is an aqueous secretion produced by the cells of the mucous glands. It serves as a covering for the mucous membranes. Mucus is mainly composed of water, which is the mucin secretion.

It is an important element of the epithelial lining fluid, the airway surface liquid, which is the lining of the respiratory tract. Mucus helps to protect the lungs during breathing by trapping foreign particles and infectious agents like dust, allergens, virus, bacteria, etc.

The human body always tends to produce more mucus in order to protect and prevent the airway tissues from drying out. Thus, there is a continuous production of mucus in the respiratory system.

When foreign objects get trapped by the mucus, the mucus becomes thick and changes color most of the time. This thick mucus that is usually coughed out as sputum is known as phlegm.

Mucus also plays an important role in the digestive system. The layer formed by the mucus in the small intestine and colon helps to protect the intestinal epithelial cells from bacterial infections. It also serves as a lubricant for the movement of foods through the esophagus.

Interestingly, mucus is the body's natural lubricant in females which helps during sexual intercourse. It also helps to fight against infection in the reproductive system.

Mucus and the Health of the Body

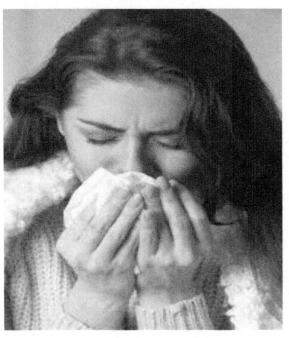

There is a continuous process of mucus production in the body, which helps to protect the body systems from infections and also provides necessary lubrication to the body.

Thus, the presence of mucus in our bodies is important. When mucus traps foreign and infectious bodies, it becomes phlegm. Phlegm and excess mucus in the body is not healthy. As the body produces up to a liter of mucus every day, it is vital to get rid of it to keep the body healthy.

Accumulation of mucus in the body is the major cause of illnesses as claimed by Dr. Sebi. So, excess mucus can be a red flag for an unhealthy state of the body.

Causes of Mucus Buildup in the Body

Just like in snails and other animals that secrete mucus, there are triggers for the production of mucus. In human beings, the major triggers are dryness and inflammation of the body. Some factors that may lead to dryness, inflammation, and other mucus secretion triggers are:

- Dry air
- Smoking
- Allergies
- Infections
- Acid reflux
- Asthma

- Low water/liquid consumption
- Medications etc.

These factors and more contribute to excess buildup of mucus in the body. The body naturally produces mucus to ensure that foreign objects (toxic and/or infectious) don't interact with the body cells. The more we have these foreign bodies, the more the body produces mucus.

When these objects get trapped by the mucus, the mucus becomes thick and builds up as phlegm.

Moreover, our body must stay lubricated for the swift movement of particles and cells in the body. Thus, dryness of the body makes the body produce more mucus, which is the liquid the body can produce naturally.

Chapter 2

ELECTRIC FOOD - ACID AND ALKALINE

Some foods and drinks change from acidic to alkaline once they are metabolized. This essentially makes them alkaline based, as once they are digested, they become alkaline. One of the most common foods in this category is citrus fruits, which contain ascorbic acid.

Citrus Fruits

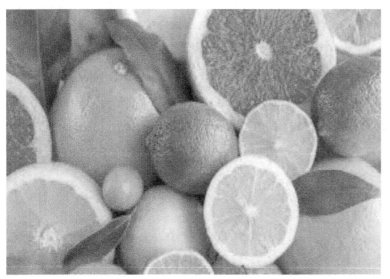

Citrus fruits may be often avoided as they are often considered acidic and sour to taste. Once they are fully digested, they effectively become alkaline in the body, with the results of increasing the pH balance to a more basic or alkaline environment. Fruits that fit into this category include lime, lemon, oranges, mandarins, tangerines, and grapefruit.

Tomatoes

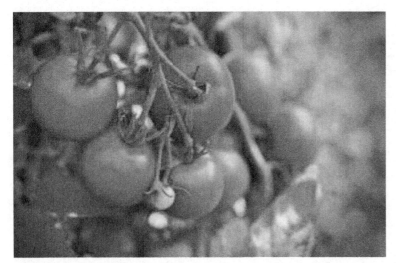

Tomatoes are another example of a fruit that becomes rich in alkaline once consumed. They are naturally acidic, and like citrus fruits, may be avoided due to their sour and sometimes strong taste. Tomatoes are best consumed in a raw state when they are digested quickly and increase the alkaline levels in the blood. When they are stewed, baked, or otherwise cooked, tomatoes increase in acidity, though are still very nutritious. If you enjoy tomatoes or cooked varieties are a regular part of your diet, incorporate both raw and cooked versions. For example, if you create pasta dishes, stew some tomatoes, and add some raw slices or cherry tomatoes as a topping to gain their benefits.

Kombucha Drinks

Kombucha is an acidic beverage that is comprised of fermented ingredients. It is typically created with a tea base (green or black tea), with added sugar for the fermentation process to form healthy bacterial cultures. There are many varieties of kombucha and recipes for flavoring and fermentation techniques. Kombucha drinks are growing in popularity in grocery stores and restaurants, though they were once considered a rare treat in upscale eateries and shops. They are available in many flavors and contain a longer shelf life than other fermented foods, such as yogurt, kimchi, and sauerkraut.

Why is kombucha beneficial for an alkaline diet? Although it is an acidic beverage, once metabolized, it becomes alkaline in the body. It is beneficial for gut health and aiding in the digestion process, which is due to the role of healthy bacteria, which also prevents infectious diseases and conditions, many of which originate in the gut. The healthy bacteria act as a barrier or protection in the stomach during the digestion process, which keeps acidic levels low to moderate. Kombucha is also high in antioxidants, which is a good defense against cancer, diabetes, and other conditions (for treatment and prevention), which is why this drink is beneficial as part of an alkaline diet.

Pineapples

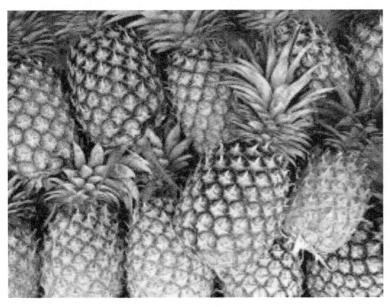

Many people will avoid pineapples because they can taste sour and cause irritation initially, though they are high in nutrients and alkalinize in the body once consumed. The benefits of pineapples include improving gut health, similarly, to fermented foods, such as yogurt and kombucha. Pineapples also reduce bloating and inflammation, which is caused by a lot of chronic and autoimmune conditions. Joint pain, arthritis, and other conditions that impact the bones and joints can be improved by the high amount of vitamin C and antioxidants in pineapples. Vitamin C improves the immunity function, which is beneficial for good health in general. If you exercise regularly and include weight or powerlifting as a part of your workout, eating pineapples and fruits high in vitamin C, fiber, and alkaline (once digested) can help your muscles recover quickly.

Apple Cider Vinegar

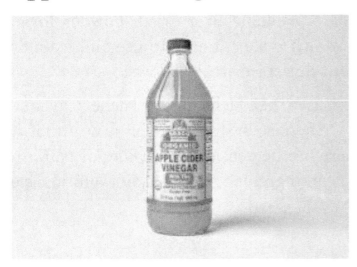

There are a lot of reported health benefits of adding apple cider vinegar to your diet, even in small amounts such as a tablespoon or two each day. This is made by mixing fermented apples with yeast and bacteria. Due to the acetic acid levels contained in it, many people avoid it altogether, as it has a pungent taste that is difficult to swallow. Diluting with water or lemon juice is one way to offset the strong taste, as well as adding to a balsamic dressing or another condiment. The benefits of apple cider vinegar work well with an alkaline diet for the following reasons:

Apple cider vinegar benefits insulin sensitivity and keeps blood sugar levels normal. While not conclusive, this effect may decrease the likelihood of developing type 2 diabetes.

Taken after a meal, it can help with the digestive process and curb overeating, which can promote weight loss and management.

It's best to consume with water or diluted with a similar drink such as tea or sparkling water to prevent the effects of the acetic acid on tooth enamel and the burning sensation on the mouth and throat if used regularly.

Hot Peppers (Including Cayenne Pepper)

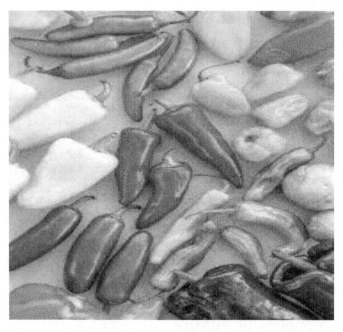

Peppers, the hot and spicy variety, and cayenne pepper, in particular, can provide a lot of health benefits. Most peppers are acidic naturally; though contain a lot of vitamin C and other nutrients that are good for your body. Cayenne pepper, specifically, becomes alkaline once it is ingested, which is a great reason to use as a seasoning in your meals, especially if you have a spicy palate. Most varieties of cayenne pepper are available in a dried, powder form, which makes it easy to use and extends the shelf life. The most important benefits of this spice are as follows:

When your body experiences pain, such as a headache or backache, cayenne provides a way of stimulating the body's response system in such a way that it diverts the sensation from the nerves, therefore decreasing the feeling of pain. In some natural remedies, cayenne is used as an ingredient to treat joint and muscle pain as a topical cream or oil.

There are some indications that cayenne pepper may aid with metabolism, which has a positive impact on weight loss. When your body produces heat, this increases the metabolism process. Cayenne pepper assists with this process, especially when enjoyed as part of a regular meal plan. While studies show that cayenne may not have consistent results in increasing metabolism over some time, it's important to note the initial benefit, as this can be a good way to start a weight loss plan.

Cayenne may suppress hunger, making you feel fuller faster and delaying the next meal or portion size. To make the most of this benefit, some people choose to take cayenne in a supplement form, such as capsules, which can usually be found in a natural health food store. If this is a supplement you want to include in your daily routine, consider finding the most natural, organic option available to ensure the maximum amount of benefits.

A lot of autoimmune conditions can be improved by changing diet, by alleviating symptoms to impact the underlying cause of the condition directly. One such condition is psoriasis, which is often treated with medications and topical creams. Capsaicin is an ingredient in cayenne, and as with creams for the treatment of joint and related pain relief, this ingredient is also used for psoriasis. Long-term benefits of reducing or possibly eliminating psoriasis by inhibiting the production of substance P in the body, which is primarily responsible for creating this condition.

Cayenne pepper is high in vitamin C and antioxidants, which can prevent and slow cancerous cell growth. Prostate, skin, and pancreatic cancers are among the types that can be prevented by cayenne pepper's nutritional ingredients.

The best benefit of cayenne pepper is how easy it is to add to most meals to enhance flavor. They are safe to eat and an excellent way to enjoy spicy food.

Chapter 3

ROLES AND FOOD PRINCIPLES

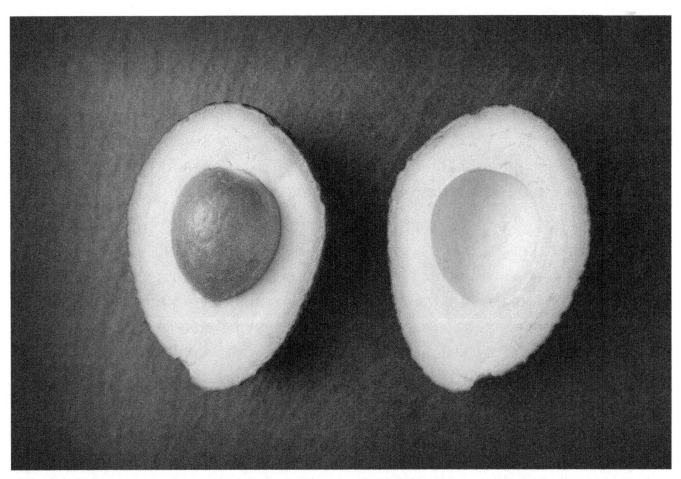

Even if you don't understand how most diets work, you know that processed meats are very bad for you when it comes to health and wellness. There have been many studies showing that processed meat can cause many diseases and illnesses. Moreover, they happen to be backed up with detailed studies to prove as such.

When following the alkaline diet, you are not allowed to eat any processed meat. It makes this diet one of the better diets when it comes to living a healthier life. Given all the benefits, you can now see how it can be an excellent idea for you to start following this diet.

Which is why they face more adversities when it comes to diseases in those specific areas; If you live in North America or a European country, then you will be facing a lot more of these diseases and problems. One of the most important things when it comes to eating processed meat is that it has been linked to an unhealthy lifestyle. Processed meat has been associated with being around people who are living an unhealthy life overall. Also, as you know, many people in the United States tend to live an unhealthy lifestyle and eat a ton of processed food. One example would be that many people who smoke cigarettes tend to eat a lot of processed meats.

Also, people who drink much alcohol will consume a lot of processed meat when they are intoxicated. This is a prevalent practice, which makes it a very unhealthy lifestyle decision. Ask yourself, when was the last time you consumed processed meat, there is a high chance that you were intoxicated the last time you consumed processed meat. Most of the time, you are eating processed meats when you are intoxicated or smoking a lot of cigarettes; moreover, people who eat a lot of processed meat tend to consume fewer fruits and vegetables.

If you're not eating the right amount of fiber and micronutrients in your diet, then there's a high chance that you're not living a healthy life overall. Basically, people who are not living a healthy life tend to consume a lot of processed meats. If you're one of them, then make sure that you rectify this situation as quickly as possible by cutting out the unhealthy things in your life which includes processed meat. Another thing that processed meat has been linked with would be chronic diseases. Eating processed meat can increase the risk of high blood pressure, heart diseases, cancer, and chronic obstructive pulmonary disease. There have been many studies showings, the people who eat this kind of meat tend to have a higher chance of attracting diseases stated above. There have also been studies done on an animal that has been consuming processed meat, and it showed that their cancer risk where bought higher when consuming processed meat as compared to when there were not.

The reason why is because processed meat contains harmful chemicals that may increase the risk of chronic diseases. There are numerous chemicals in processed meat; one of them is nitrite. This compound is one of the main reasons why your risk of cancer increases when consuming processed meat. This is the reason why the use of the compound is to preserve the red, pink color of the meat. It also helps to improve the taste of the meat and finally to get rid of any bacteria or growth in the long-term. Another reason why processed meat cannot be right for you is that it has been smoked. As we know, meat smoking is widespread when it comes to preservation.

It has often been salted and dried, to extend the shelf life of it. Once you get meat smoked in a burning wood and charcoal with dripping fat burns on a hot surface, it can cause many chemicals to form in the heat and hence making the meat very unhealthy. This is why it isn't a good idea to consume processed meats in the long-term, the way it has been made and processed makes it a terrible idea for you to consume it. There was one study done that showed when consuming processed meat every day equals smoking ten cigarettes a day in regard to the health effects you might face when consuming processed meat. This goes to show how bad processed meat can be for you. Another thing is that processed meat contains trans-fat. As you know, trans-fat is a human-made fat which has been causing many side effects on our health and wellness.

A decent amount of good fats in our diet is significant for optimal hormone production, etc. However, trans-fat can be very bad for us in the long term as it can cause many problems. One of the issues you might face when consuming trans-fat is the lowered amount of good cholesterol and the increase of bad cholesterol. Also, processed meat contains a lot of sodium, which can be very bad for us in the long-term. As you know, high amounts of sodium consumption can cause many illnesses and diseases. One of the significant things that it can cause is the risk of high blood pressure. High amounts of sodium have shown to increase blood pressure and inflammation increase, which is why it is not advisable for people to eat a lot of sodium when consuming processed meat. Processed meat can cause a lot of issues as we know by now, but one of the significant things that has been found in recent studies is that there is an increase in breast cancer.

There was one study that showed that when women consumed processed meat such as hot dogs, the risk of breast cancer went up 9%. This isn't high when you think about it, but it could still be avoided. Overall, the risk of type 2 diabetes will go up 19%, and the risk of heart disease while going up to 42% when consuming processed meat. These studies have been backed up by proper scientific studies done in a lab, which goes to show that processed meat cannot be good for health and overall well-being, which is one of the reasons why the alkaline diet does not allow you to eat meat in general, as a meat has been shown to increase the acidic levels in your body. The whole premise behind the alkaline diet is that you are not to consume foods that will raise your acidic level in your body when you have high acidic levels in your body, and there's a high chance for you to consume more bacteria. When there are more bacteria in your body, there's a high chance for you to attract more diseases and illnesses.

When it comes to attracting disease growing in your body, the bacteria like the acidic environment of your body, hence, when your body is sick, you will attract more of those diseases, and it will be more likely for you to grow them when your body is acidic. One of the most acidic things you can consume would be the use of processed meats. As you know, processed meats can cause many issues. If you're looking to follow the alkaline diet and then there's no chance in hell that you're going to be eating any processed meat. Even if you're someone looking to better your health, the first thing you need to do is cut out any processed meats that you think you're going to eat.

We can tell you what you should do and should not do, but as you can tell by the evidence that processed meat is not the answer when it comes to living a healthier life. More often than not, many of your consuming processed meat, and you don't even know it. Did you know that meats that are not organic and have been cut mechanically are also considered processed meats? These meats have been cut in a way that can cause many issues. Unfortunately, our system has made everything unhealthy when it comes to consuming food.

Chapter 4

WHAT TO EXPECT FROM THE DETOX

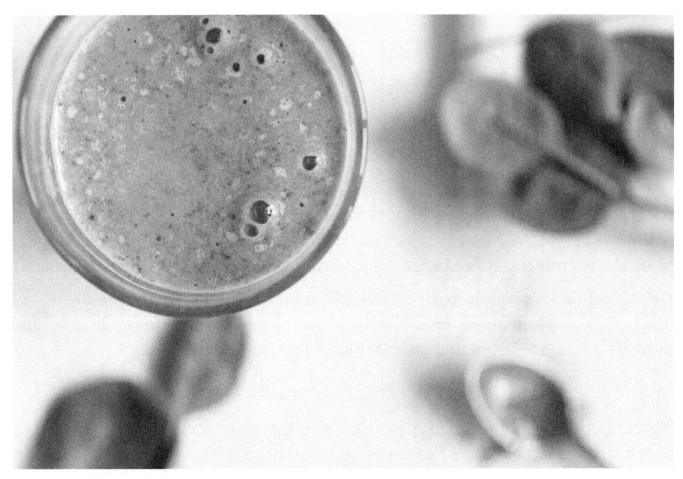

Detoxification is necessary when the body's natural detoxification organs become weak. This occurs as a result of prolonging the impact of stress, illness, poor health habit, improper diet, sedentary lifestyles, overconsumption of foods, exposure to environmental toxic substances, exposure to industrial by-products...and more.

A countless number of the toxic substances are opened to metabolic conversion or deactivation in the body and safely removed out of the body. But, when the body is loaded with environmental chemicals or when its detox organ (Liver) is not functioning well, toxins accumulate in fatty tissues and other body tissues.

Visible symptoms of this accumulation are chronic inflammation, constipation, fatigue, body odor, and overweight.

Some other dangerous effects are suppressed immune function, endocrine, and sexual dysfunction both in males and females, reduced male fertility, diabetes, increased risk for cardiovascular and liver disease.

Some chemicals found in skincare products (like Parabens) are associated with some hormones, accumulate in breast tissue, and excite the spread of human breast cancer cells.

For example, most individual's digestive systems that turn out to be unable to digest food properly; take place as a result of prolonging overconsumption of foods that are high in fats, processed foods, and low fiber foods. When this happens, food cannot move through the digestive tract and produce toxic by-products. This condition is called toxic colon syndrome or intestinal toxemia.

Detoxification is very important for individuals that have chronic health conditions such as Depression, Diabetes, Mental illness, Obesity, Cancer, Digestive disorder, Asthma, Allergies, Anxiety, Headache, High cholesterol, Arthritis, Low blood sugar level, Heart problems, Chronic fatigue syndrome, Fibromyalgia...and many others.

Detoxification is also important for individuals whose health problems are initiated by environmental conditions and for those suffering from allergies and immune deficiency issues that orthodox medicine cannot manage.

What Are the Phases of Detoxification?

As you undergo the process of detoxification, there are three major phases your body will encounter in order to achieve an accurate cure. These phases are:

Purification: in this process, you are expected to take in diets that are readily capable of detoxifying your body. This means that the diets you have to take in should be composed of detoxifying components. In this phase, you should endeavor to eat foods that are healthy and not unhealthy diets.

Restructuring/ reformation: at this phase, the body begins to adjust itself and encourages reformation. The whole system brings itself together to become healthy again.

Maintenance of good health: at this phase, the whole system interprets the information provided during the reformation phase and utilizes it to become perpetually healthy.

What Are the Benefits of Detoxification?

There are bundles of benefits you gain when you undergo the process of detoxification. These benefits are:

- It helps in weight loss and improves the well-being of the body.
- It helps in boosting the energy level.
- It helps in cleaning and strengthening the organs of detoxification and its passageways.
- It helps in boosting fertility in both men and women.
- It helps in improving mental functions.
- It helps in reducing fatigue.
- It helps in improving the appearance of the skin.
- It helps in the improvement of emotional wellbeing.
- It helps in improving memory.
- It helps in the enhancement of skin appearance.
- It helps in alleviating insomnia.
- It reduces the number of toxins in the body.
- It improves the circulatory system.
- It increases the body's immunity.
- It helps in improving optimal concentration.
- It helps in reducing stomach bloating.
- It provides strength for the nails and hair.
- It removes toxins from the liver.
- It helps in the improvement and strengthening of the digestive tract and system.
- It reduces the risk of diseases by improving the urinary system.

Chapter 5

7-DAY BALANCED ALKALINE DETOX DIET

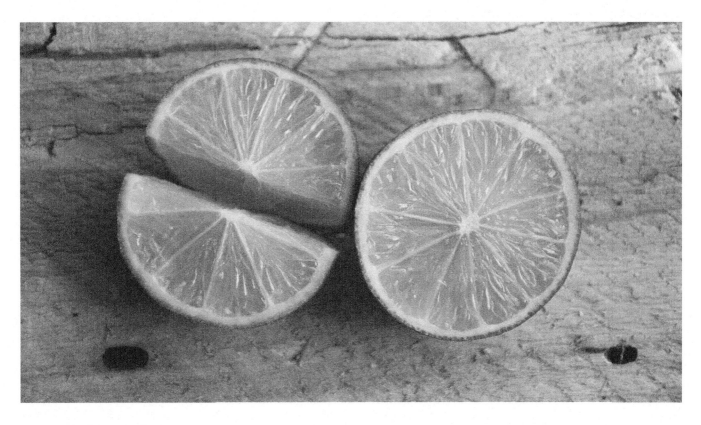

Detox Day One

Breakfast: Lime & Mint Summer Fruit Salad
Snack: Chives Chutney
Lunch: Crunchy Asparagus Spears
Dinner: Mini Turkey Meatloaves with Barbecue Sauce

Detox Day Two

Breakfast: Pumpkin Spice Quinoa
Snack: Cilantro Guacamole
Lunch: Quinoa Trail Mix Cups
Dinner: Mock Sangria

Detox Day Three

Breakfast: Jackfruit Vegetable Fry
Snack: Avocado Bites
Lunch: Oven Baked Sesame Fries
Dinner: Capriosa De Fresca

Detox Day Four

Breakfast: Banana Barley Porridge
Snack: Avocado and Radish Salsa
Lunch: Tofu & Bell Pepper Stew
Dinner: Adult Chocolate Milk with Spiced Rum

Detox Day Five

Breakfast: Zucchini Home Fries
Snack: Orange- Spiced Pumpkin Hummus
Lunch: Green Bean Casserole
Dinner: Warm Apple Delight

Detox Day Six

Breakfast: Millet Porridge
Snack: Cheesy Kale Chips
Lunch: Baked Beans
Dinner: Mock Sangria

Detox Day Seven

Breakfast: Turnip Bowl
Snack: Mini Nacho Pizzas
Lunch: Cinnamon Apple Chips with Dip
Dinner: Mixed Berry Crisp

Chapter 6

BREAKFAST RECIPES

1. Vegetable Pancakes

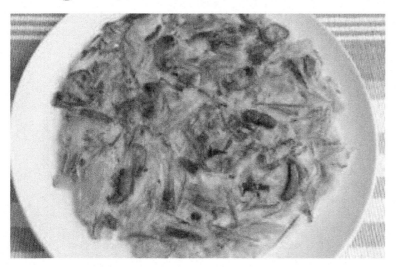

Preparation Time: 5 minutes

Cooking Time: 5 minutes

Serving: 2

Ingredients:

- ½ white onion, grated
- 1 yellow squash, roughly chopped
- 1 zucchini, peeled and chopped
- 1 zucchini, roughly chopped
- ½ teaspoon onion powder

- ¼ cup filtered water, as needed
- 1 teaspoon salt
- ¼ cup coconut flour
- 4 scallions

Directions:

1. Add the yellow squash, zucchini, zucchini, scallions, coconut flour, onion, salt, and onion powder in a food processor. Pulse until blended.
2. Add the water to the mixture to make moist but not runny. The batter will be thick.
3. Spray Pan with cooking spray and heat over medium-high heat.
4. Using an ice-cream scoop to drop batter into the pan. Use a fork to spread your mixture evenly over the pan, pressing down on the pancakes. Brown on both sides of pancakes, cooking for about 5 minutes total.
5. Serve hot and enjoy!

Nutrition: calories 254 fat 12.1 carbs 33.4 protein 6.3

2. Turnip Bowl

Preparation Time: 5 minutes

Cooking Time: 10 minutes

Serving: 2

Ingredients:

- 2 turnips, peeled and cubed
- 1 tablespoon coconut oil
- 1 red bell pepper, seeded and chopped
- 1 sweet onion, chopped
- ¼ cup mushrooms, sliced
- 4 cups kale
- 2 chive stalks, chopped
- 1 teaspoon onion powder
- 1 teaspoon onion powder
- ½ teaspoon sea salt

- ½ teaspoon bouquet garn herb blended, or other dried herbs like sage or rosemary

Directions:

1. In a bowl, combine the turnips, red bell pepper, mushrooms, kale, chives, onion, oil, onion powder, and onion powder.
2. Heat a non-stick cooking pan over medium heat, and cook the vegetables, stirring often for about 10 minutes, or until tender.
3. Serve and Enjoy!

Nutrition: calories 190, fat 2, carbs 18, protein 11

3. Millet Porridge

Preparation Time: 10 minutes

Cooking Time: 20 minutes

Serving: 2

Ingredients:

- Pinch of sea salt
- 1 tablespoon coconuts, chopped finely
- ½ cup unsweetened coconut milk
- ½ cup millet, rinsed and drained
- 1½ cups water
- 3 drops liquid stevia

Directions:

1. Sauté millet in a non-stick skillet for 3 minutes. Stir in salt and water. Let it boil then reduce the heat.
2. Cook for 15 minutes then stirs in remaining ingredients. Cook for another 4 minutes.
3. Serve with chopped nuts on top.

Nutrition: calories 219, fat 5, carbs 38, protein 6

4. Jackfruit Vegetable Fry

Preparation Time: 5 minutes

Cooking Time: 5 minutes

Serving: 6

Ingredients:

- 2 small onions, finely chopped
- 2 cups cherry tomatoes, finely chopped
- 1/8 teaspoon ground turmeric
- 1 tablespoon olive oil
- 2 red bell peppers, seeded and chopped
- 3 cups firm jackfruit, seeded and chopped
- 1/8 teaspoon cayenne pepper
- 2 tablespoons fresh basil leaves, chopped
- Salt, to taste

Directions:

1. Sauté onions and bell peppers in a greased skillet for 5 minutes. Stir in tomatoes and cook for 2 minutes.
2. Add turmeric, salt, cayenne pepper, and jackfruit. Cook for 8 minutes.
3. Garnish with basil leaves. Serve warm.

Nutrition: calories 237, fat 2, carbs 28, protein 7

5. Zucchini Pancakes

Preparation Time: 15 minutes

Cooking Time: 8 minutes

Serving: 8

Ingredients:

- 12 tablespoons water
- 6 large zucchinis, grated
- Sea salt, to taste
- 4 tablespoons ground Flax Seeds

- 2 teaspoons olive oil
- 2 jalapeño peppers, finely chopped
- ½ cup scallions, finely chopped

Directions:

1. Mix together water and flax seeds in a bowl and keep aside.
2. Heat oil in a large non-stick skillet on medium heat and add zucchini, salt, and black pepper.
3. Cook for about 3 minutes and transfer the zucchini into a large bowl. Stir in scallions and flaxseed mixture and thoroughly mix.
4. Preheat a griddle and grease it lightly with cooking spray. Pour about ¼ of the zucchini mixture into a preheated griddle and cook for about 3 minutes.
5. Flip the side carefully and cook for about 2 more minutes. Repeat with the remaining mixture in batches and serve.

Nutrition: calories 90, fat 3, carbs 22, protein 11

6. Squash Hash

Preparation Time: 2 minutes

Cooking Time: 10 minutes

Serving: 2

Ingredients:

- 1 teaspoon onion powder
- ½ cup onion, finely chopped
- 2 cups spaghetti squash
- ½ teaspoon sea salt

Directions:

1. Squeeze any extra moisture from spaghetti squash using paper towels. Place the squash into a bowl, then add the onion powder, onion, and salt. Stir to combine.
2. Spray a non-stick cooking skillet with cooking spray and place it over medium heat.

3. Add the spaghetti squash to the pan. Cook the squash for 5 minutes, untouched. Using a spatula, flip the hash browns. Cook for an additional 5 minutes or until the desired crispness is reached. Serve and Enjoy!

Nutrition: calories 212, fat 6, carbs 10, protein 10

7. Hemp Seed Porridge

Preparation Time: 5 minutes

Cooking Time: 5 minutes

Serving: 6

Ingredients:

- Hemp seed
- Stevia
- Coconut milk

Directions:

1. Combine the rice and coconut milk in a saucepan over medium heat for 5 minutes. Make sure to stir constantly.
2. Remove the pan from the heat and stir in the Stevia.
3. Divide among 6 bowls.
4. Serve and Enjoy!

Nutrition: calories 219, fat 2, carbs 18, protein 7

8. Veggie Medley

Preparation Time: 5 minutes

Cooking Time: 10 minutes

Serving:

Ingredients:

- 1 bell pepper, any color, seeded and sliced
- Juice of ½ a lime
- 2 tablespoons fresh cilantro
- ½ teaspoon cumin

- 1 teaspoon sea salt
- 1 jalapeno, chopped
- ½ cup zucchini, sliced
- 1 cup cherry tomatoes, halved
- ½ cup mushrooms, sliced
- 1 cup broccoli florets, cooked
- 1 sweet onion, chopped

Directions:

1. Spray a non-stick pan with cooking spray and place it over medium heat.
2. Add the onion, broccoli, bell pepper, tomatoes, zucchini, mushrooms, and jalapeno. Cook for 7 minutes, or until the desired doneness is reached. Stir occasionally.
3. Stir in the cumin, cilantro, and salt. Cook for 3 minutes while stirring.
4. Remove pan from heat, then add the lime juice.
5. Divide between serving plates, serve, and enjoy!

Nutrition: calories 89, fat 2, carbs 17, protein 5

9. Pumpkin Spice Quinoa

Preparation Time: 10 minutes

Cooking Time: 0 min

Serving: 2

Ingredients:

- 1 cup cooked quinoa
- 1 cup unsweetened coconut milk
- 1 large banana, mashed
- 1/4 cup pumpkin puree
- 1 teaspoon pumpkin spice
- 2 teaspoon chia seeds

Directions:

1. Mix all the ingredients in a container.
2. Seal the lid and shake well to mix.

3. Refrigerate overnight.
4. Serve.

Nutrition: calories 213, fat 6, carbs 18, protein 7

10. Zucchini Home Fries

Preparation Time: 5 minutes

Cooking Time: 20 minutes

Serving: 2

Ingredients:

- 4 medium zucchinis
- 1 teaspoon onion powder
- 1 teaspoon sea salt
- 1 red bell pepper, seeded, diced
- ½ sweet white onion, chopped
- ¼ cup vegetable broth
- ½ cup mushrooms, sliced

Directions:

1. In a medium-sized microwave-safe bowl, microwave the 4 zucchinis for about 4 minutes or until soft. Allow zucchinis to cool.
2. Add the broth into a large non-stick pan over medium heat, add the red bell pepper and onion. Sauté your vegetables for 5 minutes.
3. While the vegetables are cooking, slice your zucchinis into quarters.
4. Add the mushrooms, onion powder, salt, and zucchinis to the pan. Cook your mixture for about 10 minutes or until the zucchinis are crisp.
5. Serve and Enjoy!

Nutrition: calories 332, fat 1, carbs 34, protein 9

11. Figs & Ginger Fruit Compote

Preparation Time: 10 minutes

Cooking Time: 10 minutes

Serving: 4

Ingredients:

- 1 apple, peeled, cored, and diced
- 2 tangerines, peeled and sectioned
- ½ cup plums, dried and halved
- ½ cup figs, stemmed and quartered
- 1 packet Stevia
- ½ teaspoon cloves
- ½ teaspoon cinnamon
- 1 teaspoon ginger, fresh and grated
- 1 vanilla bean, split lengthwise, deseeded
- ¼ cup dark cherries
- 1 cup of filtered water

Directions:

1. In a saucepan, mix all of the ingredients.
2. Bring to a simmer over medium heat and cook for 10 minutes, stirring occasionally or until the fruit is tender.
3. Remove from the heat source, then let stand for 30 minutes.
4. Serve warm and Enjoy!

Nutrition: calories 102, fat 1, carbs 26, protein 1

12. Lime & Mint Summer Fruit Salad

Preparation Time: 10 minutes

Cooking Time: 0 minutes

Serving: 4

Ingredients:

- ¼ cup apple, peeled and diced
- ¼ cup grapes
- 2 tablespoons mint, fresh and chopped
- 2 tablespoons Seville orange juice, freshly squeezed
- ¼ cup strawberries
- ¼ cup peaches, peeled and diced

- ¼ cup tangerine slices
- ¼ cup cantaloupe, small bite-size pieces
- ¼ cup honeydew melon, small bite-size pieces
- ¼ cup watermelon, small bite-size pieces

Directions:

1. In a mixing bowl, combine all of the fruit.
2. Add the Seville orange juice, mint, and mix well.
3. Serve chilled and enjoy!

Nutrition: calories 150, fat 1, carbs 7, protein 2

13. Banana Barley Porridge

Preparation Time: 5 minutes

Cooking Time: 30 minutes

Serving: 2

Ingredients:

- 1 cup unsweetened coconut milk, divided
- 1 small banana, peeled and sliced
- ½ cup barley
- 3 drops liquid stevia
- ¼ cup coconuts, chopped

Directions:

1. Mix barley with half coconut milk and stevia in a bowl and mix well. Cover and refrigerate for about 6 hours.
2. Mix the barley mixture with coconut milk in a saucepan. Cook for 5 minutes on medium heat.
3. Top with chopped coconuts and banana slices. Serve.

Nutrition: calories 420, fat 3, carbs 28, protein 7

14. Zucchini Muffins

Preparation Time: 10 minutes

Cooking Time: 25 minutes

Serving: 16

Ingredients:

- 1 tablespoon ground flaxseed
- 3 tablespoons water
- ¼ cup walnut butter
- 3 small-medium over-ripe bananas
- 2 small zucchinis, grated
- ½ cup coconut milk
- 1 teaspoon vanilla extract
- 2 cups coconut flour
- 1 tablespoon baking powder
- 1 teaspoon cinnamon
- ¼ teaspoon sea salt
- Optional add-ins:
- ¼ cup chocolate chips and/or walnuts

Directions:

1. Set your oven to 375 degrees F. Grease a muffin tray with cooking spray. Mix flaxseed with water in a bowl.
2. Mash bananas in a glass bowl and stir in all the remaining ingredients. Mix well and divide the mixture into the muffin tray.
3. Bake for 25 minutes. Serve.

Nutrition: calories 170, fat 4, carbs 13, protein 1

15. Millet Porridge

Preparation Time: 10 minutes

Cooking Time: 20 minutes

Serving: 2

Ingredients:

- Pinch of sea salt
- 1 tablespoon coconuts, chopped finely
- ½ cup unsweetened coconut milk
- ½ cup millet, rinsed and drained
- 1½ cups water
- 3 drops liquid stevia

Directions:

1. Sauté millet in a non-stick skillet for 3 minutes. Stir in salt and water. Let it boil then reduce the heat.
2. Cook for 15 minutes then stirs in remaining ingredients. Cook for another 4 minutes.
3. Serve with chopped nuts on top.

Nutrition: calories 219, fat 2, carbs 8, protein 6

16. Jackfruit Vegetable Fry

Preparation Time: 5 minutes

Cooking Time: 5 minutes

Serving: 6

Ingredients:

- 2 small onions, finely chopped
- 2 cups cherry tomatoes, finely chopped
- 1/8 teaspoon ground turmeric
- 1 tablespoon olive oil
- 2 red bell peppers, seeded and chopped
- 3 cups firm jackfruit, seeded and chopped
- 1/8 teaspoon cayenne pepper
- 2 tablespoons fresh basil leaves, chopped
- Salt, to taste

Directions:

1. Sauté onions and bell peppers in a greased skillet for 5 minutes. Stir in tomatoes and cook for 2 minutes.
2. Add turmeric, salt, cayenne pepper, and jackfruit. Cook for 8 minutes.
3. Garnish with basil leaves. Serve warm.

Nutrition: calories 236, fat 2, carbs 10, protein 7

17. Zucchini Pancakes

Preparation Time: 15 minutes

Cooking Time: 8 minutes

Serving: *8*

Ingredients:

- 12 tablespoons water
- 6 large zucchinis, grated
- Sea salt, to taste
- 4 tablespoons ground Flax Seeds
- 2 teaspoons olive oil
- 2 jalapeño peppers, finely chopped
- ½ cup scallions, finely chopped

Directions:

1. Mix together water and flax seeds in a bowl and keep aside.
2. Heat oil in a large non-stick skillet on medium heat and add zucchini, salt, and black pepper.
3. Cook for about 3 minutes and transfer the zucchini into a large bowl. Stir in scallions and flaxseed mixture and thoroughly mix.
4. Preheat a griddle and grease it lightly with cooking spray. Pour about ¼ of the zucchini mixture into a preheated griddle and cook for about 3 minutes.
5. Flip the side carefully and cook for about 2 more minutes. Repeat with the remaining mixture in batches and serve.

Nutrition: calories 132, fat 3, carbs 9, protein 4

18. Squash Hash

Preparation Time: 2 minutes

Cooking Time: 10 minutes

Serving: 2

Ingredients:

- 1 teaspoon onion powder
- ½ cup onion, finely chopped
- 2 cups spaghetti squash
- ½ teaspoon sea salt

Directions:

1. Squeeze any extra moisture from spaghetti squash using paper towels. Place the squash into a bowl, then add the onion powder, onion, and salt. Stir to combine.
2. Spray a non-stick cooking skillet with cooking spray and place it over medium heat.
3. Add the spaghetti squash to the pan. Cook the squash for 5 minutes, untouched. Using a spatula, flip the hash browns. Cook for an additional 5 minutes or until the desired crispness is reached. Serve and Enjoy!

Nutrition: calories 180, fat 2, carbs 8, protein 1

19. Veggie Medley

Preparation Time: 5 minutes

Cooking Time: 10 minutes

Serving: 2

Ingredients:

- 1 bell pepper, any color, seeded and sliced
- Juice of ½ a lime
- 2 tablespoons fresh cilantro
- ½ teaspoon cumin
- 1 teaspoon sea salt

- 1 jalapeno, chopped
- ½ cup zucchini, sliced
- 1 cup cherry tomatoes, halved
- ½ cup mushrooms, sliced
- 1 cup broccoli florets, cooked
- 1 sweet onion, chopped

Directions:

1. Spray a non-stick pan with cooking spray and place it over medium heat.
2. Add the onion, broccoli, bell pepper, tomatoes, zucchini, mushrooms, and jalapeno. Cook for 7 minutes, or until the desired doneness is reached. Stir occasionally.
3. Stir in the cumin, cilantro, and salt. Cook for 3 minutes while stirring.
4. Remove pan from heat, then add the lime juice.
5. Divide between serving plates, serve, and enjoy!

Nutrition: calories 90, fat 2, carbs 16, protein 4

20. Pumpkin Spice Quinoa

Preparation Time: 10 minutes

Cooking Time: 0 min

Serving: 2

Ingredients:

- 1 cup cooked quinoa
- 1 cup unsweetened coconut milk
- 1 large banana, mashed
- 1/4 cup pumpkin puree
- 1 teaspoon pumpkin spice
- 2 teaspoon chia seeds

Directions:

1. Mix all the ingredients in a container.
2. Seal the lid and shake well to mix.
3. Refrigerate overnight.

4. Serve.

Nutrition: calories 216, fat 2, carbs 18, protein 9

21. Zucchini Home Fries

Preparation Time: 5 minutes

Cooking Time: 20 minutes

Serving: 2

Ingredients:

- 4 medium zucchinis
- 1 teaspoon onion powder
- 1 teaspoon sea salt
- 1 red bell pepper, seeded, diced
- ½ sweet white onion, chopped
- ¼ cup vegetable broth
- ½ cup mushrooms, sliced

Directions:

1. In a medium-sized microwave-safe bowl, microwave the 4 zucchinis for about 4 minutes or until soft. Allow zucchinis to cool.
2. Add the broth into a large non-stick pan over medium heat, add the red bell pepper and onion. Sauté your vegetables for 5 minutes.
3. While the vegetables are cooking, slice your zucchinis into quarters.
4. Add the mushrooms, onion powder, salt, and zucchinis to the pan. Cook your mixture for about 10 minutes or until the zucchinis are crisp.
5. Serve and Enjoy!

Nutrition: calories 321, fat 2, carbs 28, protein 11

22. Figs & Ginger Fruit Compote

Preparation Time: 10 minutes

Cooking Time: 10 minutes

Serving: 4

Ingredients:

- 1 apple, peeled, cored, and diced
- 2 tangerines, peeled and sectioned
- ½ cup plums, dried and halved
- ½ cup figs, stemmed and quartered
- 1 packet stevia
- ½ teaspoon cloves
- ½ teaspoon cinnamon
- 1 teaspoon ginger, fresh and grated
- 1 vanilla bean, split lengthwise, deseeded
- ¼ cup dark cherries
- 1 cup of filtered water

Directions:

1. In a saucepan, mix all of the ingredients.
2. Bring to a simmer over medium heat and cook for 10 minutes, stirring occasionally or until the fruit is tender.
3. Remove from the heat source, then let stand for 30 minutes.
4. Serve warm and Enjoy!

Nutrition: calories 130, fat 1, carbs 26, protein 1

23. Lime & Mint Summer Fruit Salad

Preparation Time: 10 minutes

Cooking Time: 0 minutes

Serving: 4

Ingredients:

- ¼ cup apple, peeled and diced
- ¼ cup grapes
- 2 tablespoons mint, fresh and chopped
- 2 tablespoons Seville orange juice, freshly squeezed
- ¼ cup strawberries
- ¼ cup peaches, peeled and diced

- ¼ cup tangerine slices
- ¼ cup cantaloupe, small bite-size pieces
- ¼ cup honeydew melon, small bite-size pieces
- ¼ cup watermelon, small bite-size pieces

Directions:

1. In a mixing bowl, combine all of the fruit.
2. Add the Seville orange juice, mint, and mix well.
3. Serve chilled and enjoy!

Nutrition: calories 86, fat 0, carbs 7, protein 1

24. Dr. Sebi Granola

Preparation Time: 2 minutes

Cooking Time: 15 minutes

Serving: 4

Ingredients:

- 1 cup slivered coconuts
- 1 cup flaked unsweetened coconut
- ½ cup raisins
- ½ cup flaxseed
- ½ teaspoon nutmeg
- ½ teaspoon cinnamon
- ¼ teaspoon ginger
- ¼ teaspoon sea salt
- ½ cup unsweetened dried pineapple pieces
- ¼ cup coconut oil

Directions:

1. Preheat your oven to 350° Fahrenheit.
2. In a bowl, combine the coconut, flaxseed, coconuts, raisins, ginger, cinnamon, nutmeg, vanilla bean seeds, salt, and coconut oil. Mix until well combined.

3. Spread the mix on a baking sheet and bake for 15 minutes, occasionally stirring, until golden brown.
4. Remove from your oven and cool, without stirring.
5. Once cooled, stir in the pineapple pieces.
6. Store in an airtight container.

Nutrition: calories 219, fat 1, carbs 18, protein 1

25. Vegetable Pancakes

Preparation Time: 5 minutes

Cooking Time: 5 minutes

Serving: 2

Ingredients:

- ½ white onion, grated
- 1 yellow squash, roughly chopped
- 1 zucchini, peeled and chopped
- 1 zucchini, roughly chopped
- ½ teaspoon onion powder
- ¼ cup filtered water, as needed
- 1 teaspoon salt
- ¼ cup coconut flour
- 4 scallions

Directions:

1. Add the yellow squash, zucchini, zucchini, scallions, coconut flour, onion, salt, and onion powder in a food processor. Pulse until blended.
2. Add the water to the mixture to make moist but not runny. The batter will be thick.
3. Spray Pan with cooking spray and heat over medium-high heat.
4. Using an ice-cream scoop to drop batter into the pan. Use a fork to spread your mixture evenly over the pan, pressing down on the pancakes. Brown on both sides of pancakes, cooking for about 5 minutes total.
5. Serve hot and Enjoy!

Nutrition: calories 140, fat 1, carbs 8, protein 1

26. Turnip Bowl

Preparation Time: 5 minutes

Cooking Time: 10 minutes

Serving: 2

Ingredients:

- 2 turnips, peeled and cubed
- 1 tablespoon coconut oil
- 1 red bell pepper, seeded and chopped
- 1 sweet onion, chopped
- ¼ cup mushrooms, sliced
- 4 cups kale
- 2 chive stalks, chopped
- 1 teaspoon onion powder
- 1 teaspoon onion powder
- ½ teaspoon sea salt
- ½ teaspoon Bouquet Garn herb blended, or other dried herbs like sage or rosemary

Directions:

1. In a bowl, combine the turnips, red bell pepper, mushrooms, kale, chives, onion, oil, onion powder, and onion powder.
2. Heat a non-stick cooking pan over medium heat, and cook the vegetables, stirring often for about 10 minutes, or until tender.
3. Serve and Enjoy!

Nutrition: calories 211, fat 1, carbs 9, protein 1

Chapter 7

SMOOTHIES

27. Pineapple, Banana & Spinach Smoothie

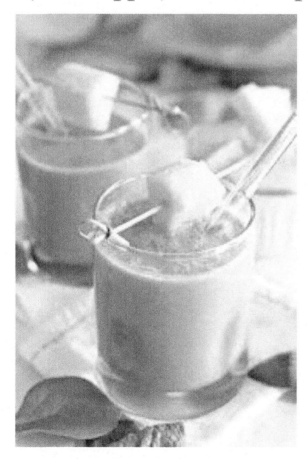

Preparation Time: 10 Minutes

Cooking time: 0 minute

Servings: 1

Ingredients:

- ½ cup almond milk
- ¼ cup soy yogurt
- 1 cup spinach
- 1 cup banana
- 1 cup pineapple chunks
- 1 tbsp. chia seeds

Directions:

1. Add all the ingredients to a blender.
2. Blend until smooth.
3. Chill in the refrigerator before serving.

Nutrition: calories 153, fat 1, carbs 8, protein 1

28. Kale & Avocado Smoothie

Preparation Time: 10 Minutes

Cooking time: 0 minute

Servings: 1

Ingredients:

- 1 ripe banana
- 1 cup kale
- 1 cup almond milk
- ¼ avocado
- 1 tbsp. chia seeds
- 2 tsp. honey
- 1 cup ice cubes

Direction:

1. Blend all the ingredients until smooth.

Nutrition: calories 133, fat 1, carbs 9, protein 1

29. Coconut & Strawberry Smoothie

Preparation Time: 10 Minutes

Cooking Time: 0 minutes

Serves: 1

Ingredients:

- 1 Cup Strawberries, Frozen & Thawed Slightly
- 1 Ripe Banana, Sliced & Frozen
- ½ Cup Coconut Milk, Light
- ½ Cup Vegan Yogurt
- 1 Tablespoon Chia Seeds
- 1 Teaspoon Lime juice, Fresh
- 4 Ice Cubes

Directions:

1. Blend everything together until smooth and serve immediately.

Nutrition: calories 210, fat 2, carbs 7, protein 9

30. Pumpkin Chia Smoothie

Preparation Time: 5 Minutes

Cooking Time: 0 minutes

Servings: 1

Ingredients:

- 3 Tablespoons Pumpkin Puree
- 1 Tablespoon MCT Oil
- ¾ Cup Coconut Milk, Full Fat
- ½ Avocado, Fresh
- 1 Teaspoon Vanilla, Pure
- ½ Teaspoon Pumpkin Pie Spice

Directions:

1. Combine all ingredients together until blended.

Nutrition: calories 188, fat 1, carbs 9, protein 1

31. Cantaloupe Smoothie Bowl

Preparation Time: 5 Minutes

Cooking Time: 0 minutes

Servings: 2

Ingredients:

- ¾ cup carrot juice
- 4 cups cantaloupe, frozen & cubed
- Melon balls or berries to serve
- Pinch sea salt

Directions:

1. Blend everything together until smooth.

Nutrition: calories 105, fat 1, carbs 3, protein 9

32. Berry & Cauliflower Smoothie

Preparation Time: 10 Minutes

Cooking Time: 0 minutes

Servings: 2

Ingredients:

- 1 Cup Riced Cauliflower, Frozen
- 1 Cup Banana, Sliced & Frozen
- ½ Cup Mixed Berries, Frozen
- 2 Cups Almond Milk, Unsweetened
- 2 Teaspoons Maple syrup, Pure & Optional

Directions:

1. Blend until mixed well.

Nutrition: calories 122, fat 1, carbs 4, protein 10

33. Green Mango Smoothie

Preparation Time: 5 Minutes

Cooking Time: 0 minutes

Servings: 1

Ingredients:

- 2 Cups Spinach
- 1-2 Cups Coconut Water
- 2 Mangos, Ripe, Peeled & Diced

Directions:

1. Blend everything together until smooth.

Nutrition: calories 120, fat 1, carbs 5, protein 8

34. Chia Seed Smoothie

Preparation Time: 5 Minutes

Cooking Time: 0 minutes

Servings: 3

Ingredients:

- ¼ Teaspoon Cinnamon
- 1 Tablespoon Ginger, Fresh & Grated
- Pinch Cardamom
- 1 Tablespoon Chia Seeds
- 2 Medjool Dates, Pitted
- 1 Cup Alfalfa Sprouts
- 1 Cup Water
- 1 Banana
- ½ Cup Coconut Milk, Unsweetened

Directions:

1. Blend everything together until smooth.

35. Mango Smoothie

Preparation Time: 5 Minutes

Cooking Time: 0 minutes

Servings: 3

Ingredients:

- 1 Carrot, Peeled & Chopped
- 1 Cup Strawberries
- 1 Cup Water
- 1 Cup Peaches, Chopped
- 1 Banana, Frozen & sliced
- 1 Cup Mango, Chopped

Directions:

1. Blend everything together until smooth.

Nutrition: calories 221, fat 1, carbs 5, protein 4

36. Spinach Peach Banana Smoothie

Preparation Time: 10 minutes

Cooking Time: 0 minutes

Servings: 2

Ingredients:

- 1 cup baby spinach
- 2 cups coconut water
- 1 tablespoon agave syrup
- 2 ripe bananas
- 2 ripe peaches, pitted and chopped

Directions:

1. Add all ingredients to the blender and blend until smooth and creamy.
2. Serve immediately and enjoy.

Nutrition: calories 163, fat 1, carbs 4, protein 6

37. Salty Green Smoothie

Preparation Time: 10 minutes

Cooking Time: 0 minutes

Servings: 2

Ingredients:

- 1 cup ice cubes
- 1/4 tablespoon liquid aminos
- 1 and 1/2 tablespoon sea salt
- 2 limes, peeled and quartered
- 1 avocado, pitted and peeled
- 1 cup kale leaves
- 1 cucumber, chopped
- 2 cups tomato, chopped
- 1/4 cup water

Directions:

1. Add all ingredients to the blender and blend until smooth and creamy.
2. Serve immediately and enjoy.

Nutrition: calories 108, fat 1, carbs 1, protein 4

38. Watermelon Strawberry Smoothie

Preparation Time: 10 minutes

Cooking Time: 0 minutes

Servings: 2

Ingredients:

- 1 cup coconut milk yogurt
- 1/2 cup strawberries
- 2 cups fresh watermelon
- 1 banana

Directions:

1. Toss in all your ingredients into your blender then process until smooth.

2. Serve and Enjoy.

Nutrition: calories 160, fat 1, carbs 3, protein 4

39. Watermelon Kale Smoothie

Preparation Time: 10 minutes

Cooking Time: 0 minutes

Servings: 2

Ingredients:

- 8 oz water
- 1 orange, peeled
- 3 cups kale, chopped
- 1 banana, peeled
- 2 cups watermelon, chopped
- 1 celery, chopped

Directions:

1. Add all ingredients to the blender and blend until smooth and creamy.
2. Serve immediately and Enjoy.

Nutrition: calories 122, fat 1, carbs 5, protein 1

40. Mix Berry Watermelon Smoothie

Preparation Time: 10 minutes

Cooking Time: 0 minutes

Servings: 2

Ingredients:

- 1 cup alkaline water
- 2 fresh lemon juices
- 1/4 cup fresh mint leaves
- 1 and 1/2 cup mixed berries
- 2 cups watermelon

Directions:

1. Toss in all your ingredients into your blender then process until smooth. Serve immediately and Enjoy.

Nutrition: calories 188, fat 1, carbs 2, protein 1

41. Healthy Green Smoothie

Preparation Time: 10 minutes

Cooking Time: 0 minutes

Servings: 3

Ingredients:

- 1 cup water
- 1 fresh lemon, peeled
- 1 avocado
- 1 cucumber, peeled
- 1 cup spinach
- 1 cup ice cubes

Directions:

1. Add all ingredients to the blender and blend until smooth and creamy.
2. Serve immediately and enjoy.

Nutrition: Calories: 160, Fat 13, Carbs: 12, Protein 2

42. Apple Spinach Cucumber Smoothie

Preparation Time: 10 minutes

Cooking Time: 0 minutes

Servings: 1

Ingredients:

- 3/4 cup water
- 1/2 green apple, diced
- 3/4 cup spinach
- 1/2 cucumber

Directions:

1. Add all ingredients to the blender and blend until smooth and creamy.
2. Serve immediately and enjoy.

Nutrition: calories 90, fat 1, carbs 21, protein 1

43. Refreshing Lime Smoothie

Preparation Time: 10 minutes

Cooking Time: 0 minutes

Servings: 2

Ingredients:

- 1 cup ice cubes
- 20 drops liquid stevia
- 2 fresh lime, peeled and halved
- 1 tablespoon lime zest, grated
- 1/2 cucumber, chopped
- 1 avocado, pitted and peeled
- 2 cups spinach
- 1 tablespoon creamed coconut
- 3/4 cup coconut water

Directions:

1. Add all ingredients to the blender and blend until smooth and creamy.
2. Serve immediately and enjoy.

Nutrition: calories 312, fat 3, carbs 28, protein 4

44. Broccoli Green Smoothie

Preparation Time: 10 minutes

Cooking Time: 0 minutes

Servings: 2

Ingredients:

- 1 celery, peeled and chopped
- 1 lemon, peeled
- 1 apple, diced
- 1 banana
- 1 cup spinach
- 1/2 cup broccoli

Directions:

1. Add all ingredients to the blender and blend until smooth and creamy.
2. Serve immediately and enjoy.

Nutrition: calories 121, fat 1, carbs 18, protein 1

45. Healthy Vegetable Smoothie

Preparation Time: 10 minutes

Cooking Time: 0 minutes

Servings: 2

Ingredients:

- 1 cup ice cubes
- 2 cups fresh spinach
- 2 celery stalks
- 1/2 cup fresh parsley
- 1 cucumber
- 1 lemon juice
- 1 avocado

Directions:

1. Add all ingredients to the blender and blend until smooth and creamy.
2. Serve immediately and enjoy.

Nutrition: calories 210, fat 3, carbs 17, protein 11

46. Refreshing Green Smoothie

Preparation Time: 10 minutes

Cooking Time: 0 minutes

Servings: 2

Ingredients:

- 1 cup ice cubes
- 1/2 lemon juice
- 1/2 cucumber, chopped
- 1/4 cup parsley
- 1 cup spinach
- 1/2 cup water
- 1/4 cup peaches, sliced
- 1 banana

Directions:

1. Add all ingredients to the blender and blend until smooth and creamy.
2. Serve immediately and enjoy.

Nutrition: calories 90, fat 1, carbs 20, protein

47. Sweet Green Smoothie

Preparation Time: 10 minutes

Cooking Time: 0 minutes

Servings: 1

Ingredients:

- 2 tablespoons flax seeds
- 1/2 cup wheatgrass
- 1 mango
- 1 cup pomegranate juice

Directions:

1. Add all ingredients to the blender and blend until smooth and creamy.
2. Serve immediately and enjoy.

Nutrition: calories 177, fat 1, carbs 21, protein 5

48. Avocado Mango Smoothie

Preparation Time: 10 minutes

Cooking Time: 0 minutes

Servings: 2

Ingredients:

- 1 cup ice cubes
- 1/2 cup mango
- 1/2 avocado
- 1 tablespoon ginger
- 3 kale leaves
- 1 cup coconut water

Directions:

1. Toss in all your ingredients into your blender then process until smooth.
2. Serve and Enjoy.

Nutrition: calories 290, fat 3, carbs 18, protein 11

49. Super Healthy Green Smoothie

Preparation Time: 10 minutes

Cooking Time: 0 minutes

Servings: 2

Ingredients:

- 1 teaspoon spirulina powder
- 1 cup coconut water
- 2 cups mixed greens
- 1 tablespoon ginger
- 4 tablespoon lemon juice
- 2 celery stalks
- 1 cup cucumber, chopped
- 1 green pear, core removed

- 1 banana

Directions:

1. Add all ingredients to the blender and blend until smooth and creamy.
2. Serve immediately and enjoy.

Nutrition: calories 161, fat 1, carbs 19, protein 7

50. Spinach Coconut Smoothie

Preparation Time: 10 minutes

Cooking Time: 0 minutes

Servings: 2

Ingredients:

- 2 tablespoons unsweetened coconut flakes
- 2 cups fresh pineapple
- 1/2 cup coconut water
- 1 and 1/2 cups coconut milk
- 2 cups fresh spinach

Directions:

1. Add all ingredients to the blender and blend until smooth and creamy.
2. Serve immediately and enjoy.

Nutrition: calories 290, fat 1, carbs 22, protein 8

51. Pear Kale Smoothie

Preparation Time: 10 minutes

Cooking Time: 0 minutes

Servings: 2

Ingredients:

- 1 cup apple juice
- 1 cup water
- 1/4 cup mint leaves
- 2 cups kale

- 1 ripe pear, cored and chopped

Directions:

1. Add all ingredients to the blender and blend until smooth and creamy.
2. Serve immediately and enjoy.

Nutrition: calories 130, fat 1, carbs 18, protein 3

52. Banana Peach Smoothie

Preparation Time: 10 minutes

Cooking Time: 0 minutes

Servings: 2

Ingredients:

- 1 cup coconut water
- 1 teaspoon agave syrup
- 1 and 1/4 oz spinach
- 1 banana
- 1 ripe peach

Directions:

1. Add all ingredients to the blender and blend until smooth and creamy.
2. Serve immediately and enjoy.

Nutrition: calories 120, fat 2, carbs 28, protein 10

53. Refreshing Alkaline Smoothie

Preparation Time: 10 minutes

Cooking Time: 0 minutes

Servings: 2

Ingredients:

- 1/2 cup ice cubes
- 1 tbsp ginger
- 1/4 cup fresh mint leaves
- 1/2 cup parsley

- 1 cucumber, chopped
- 1 lemon juice
- 1 cup water
- 4 cups baby spinach
- 1 avocado

Directions:

1. Add all ingredients to the blender and blend until smooth and creamy.
2. Serve immediately and enjoy.

Nutrition: calories 267, fat 1, carbs 10, protein 4

54. Coconut Celery Smoothie

Preparation Time: 10 minutes

Cooking Time: 0 minutes

Servings: 2

Ingredients:

- 3 celeries, shredded
- 1 teaspoon ground cinnamon
- 1/2 banana
- 1 scoop protein powder
- 1 tablespoon coconut butter
- 1 cup unsweetened coconut milk

Directions:

1. Add all ingredients to the blender and blend until smooth and creamy.
2. Serve immediately and enjoy.

Nutrition: calories 319, fat 1, carbs 18, protein 9

55. Blueberry Coconut Smoothie

Preparation Time: 10 minutes

Cooking Time: 0 minutes

Servings: 1

Ingredients:

- 1 tablespoon hemp seeds
- 1/2 cup blueberries
- 1 teaspoon ground cinnamon
- 1/2 banana
- 1 scoop protein powder
- 1 tablespoon coconut butter
- 1 cup unsweetened coconut milk

Directions:

1. Add all ingredients to the blender and blend until smooth and creamy.
2. Serve immediately and enjoy.

Nutrition: calories 211, fat 1, carbs 19, protein 8

56. Kiwi Cucumber Boosting Smoothie

Preparation Time: 10 minutes

Cooking Time: 0 minutes

Servings: 1

Ingredients:

- 1 cup spinach
- 1 cup ice cubes
- 1 kiwi fruit
- 1/2 banana
- 1/4 cucumber
- 1/4 cup coconut milk

Directions:

1. Add all ingredients to the blender and blend until smooth and creamy.
2. Serve immediately and enjoy.

Nutrition: calories 255, fat 1, carbs 20, protein 6

57. Spinach Protein Smoothie

Preparation Time: 10 minutes

Cooking Time: 0 minutes

Servings: 2

Ingredients:

*   1 and 1/2 cups unsweetened coconut milk
*   1/2 cup yogurt
*   1/2 teaspoon cinnamon
*   1 tablespoon protein powder
*   1/2 banana
*   2 cups spinach

Directions:

1. Toss in all your ingredients into your blender then process until smooth.
2. Serve and enjoy.

Nutrition: calories 390, fat 1, carbs 24, protein 11

58. Tropical Smoothie

Preparation Time: 10 minutes

Cooking Time: 0 minutes

Servings: 1

Ingredients:

*   1/4 cup coconut water
*   1/2 cup yogurt
*   1 tablespoon honey
*   2 tablespoons shredded coconut

- 1/2 cup mango
- 1/2 cup pineapple
- 1 and 1/2 cup spinach

Directions:

1. Add all ingredients to the blender and blend until smooth and creamy.
2. Serve immediately and enjoy.

Nutrition: calories 219, fat 1, carbs 9, protein 4

59. Berry Kale Smoothie

Preparation Time: 10 minutes

Cooking Time: 0 minutes

Servings: 1

Ingredients:

- 1 cup orange juice
- 1/2 cup yogurt
- 1 banana
- 1/4 cup raspberries
- 1/2 cup strawberries
- 1 cup kale

Directions:

1. Add all ingredients to the blender and blend until smooth and creamy.
2. Serve immediately and enjoy.

Nutrition: calories 312, fat 2, carbs 18, protein 12

60. Basil Kale Strawberry Smoothie

Preparation Time: 10 minutes

Cooking Time: 0 minutes

Servings: 2

Ingredients:

- 1 and 1/2 cups unsweetened coconut milk
- 1 tablespoon flax seeds
- 1/4 cup basil
- 3 strawberries
- 1/2 banana
- 1 cup kale

Directions:

1. Add all ingredients to the blender and blend until smooth and creamy.
2. Serve immediately and enjoy.

Nutrition: calories 203, fat 3, carbs 28, protein 5

61. Chia Strawberry Smoothie

Preparation Time: 10 minutes

Cooking Time: 0 minutes

Servings: 2

Ingredients:

- 4 drops liquid stevia
- 1/2 lemon juice
- 1/2 small beetroot, chopped
- 1 cup strawberries
- 4 romaine lettuce leaves, chopped
- 2 celery stalks, chopped
- 2 tablespoons chia seeds
- 1 cup coconut water

Directions:

1. Add all ingredients to the blender and blend until smooth and creamy.
2. Serve immediately and enjoy.

Nutrition: calories 90, fat 3, carbs 15, protein 3

62. Strawberry Banana Smoothie

Preparation Time: 10 minutes

Cooking Time: 0 minutes

Servings: 1

Ingredients:

- 1 cup unsweetened coconut milk
- 1 banana
- 1/2 cup strawberries

Directions:

1. Add all ingredients to the blender and blend until smooth and creamy.
2. Serve immediately and enjoy.

Nutrition: calories 85, fat 3, carbs 18, protein 11

63. Easy Mango Lassi

Preparation Time: 10 minutes

Cooking Time: 0 minutes

Servings: 4

Ingredients

- 2 cups plain whole-milk yogurt
- 1 cup milk
- 3 mangoes - peeled, seeded, and chopped
- 4 tsps. white sugar, or to taste
- 1/8 tsp. ground cardamom

Directions:

1. In the jar of a blender, place cardamom, white sugar, mangoes, milk, and yogurt.
2. Blend together for about 2 minutes or until smooth.
3. Chill in the refrigerator until cold, about 1 hour.
4. Serve with a small sprinkling of ground cardamom.

Nutrition: calories 220, fat 1, carbs 24, protein 4

64. Holly Goodness Smoothie

Preparation Time: 10 minutes

Cooking Time: 0 minutes

Servings: 1

Ingredients

- 1 mango - peeled, seeded, and chopped
- 1 small banana
- 1/2 cup frozen raspberries
- 1/2 cup almond milk
- 1/2 cup hemp milk
- 1 tsp. vanilla extract
- 1 tsp. chia seeds
- 1 tsp. hemp seeds
- 1 tsp. maca powder

Directions:

1. Blend together maca powder, hemp seeds, chia seeds, vanilla extract, hemp milk, almond milk, raspberries, banana, and mango using a blender until the mixture is smooth.

Nutrition: calories 380, fat 2, carbs 20, protein 11

65. Honey-mango Smoothie

Preparation Time: 10 minutes

Cooking Time: 0 minutes

Servings: 2

Ingredients:

- 1 mango - peeled, seeded, and cubed
- 1 tbsp. white sugar
- 2 tbsps. honey
- 1 cup nonfat milk
- 1 tsp. lemon juice

- 1 cup ice cubes

Directions:

1. In a blender pitcher, put sugar, honey, and mango; add lemon juice and milk, conflate till smooth. Distribute ice cubes among 2 serving glasses.
2. Put mango smoothie on ice and serve.

Nutrition: calories 310, fat 3, carbs 28, protein 3

66. Hong Kong Mango Drink

Preparation Time: 10 minutes

Cooking Time: 0 minutes

Servings: 2

Ingredients:

- 1/2 cup small pearl tapioca
- 1 mango - peeled, seeded, and diced
- 14 ice cubes
- 1/2 cup coconut milk

Directions:

1. Over high heat, boil water.
2. When the water is boiling, mix in the tapioca pearls then boil again.
3. Uncover while cooking the tapioca pearls for 10 minutes, mixing from time to time. Put the cover back then take off heat, let it rest for half an hour.
4. In a colander placed in the sink, drain well; cover then chill.
5. In a blender, blend ice and mango till smooth. In 2 tall glasses, distribute chilled tapioca pearls; pour the mango mixture on top then pour on top of each with a quarter cup coconut milk.

Nutrition: calories 324, fat 2, carbs 21, protein 9

67. Jack-o'-lantern Smoothie Bowl

Preparation Time: 10 minutes

Cooking Time: 0 minutes

Servings: 1

Ingredients:

- 1 cup frozen mango chunks
- ¾ cup reduced-fat plain Greek yogurt
- ¼ cup reduced-fat milk
- 1 tsp. vanilla extract
- 1 strawberry, hulled and halved
- 1 tsp. chia seeds

Directions:

1. In a blender, combine vanilla, milk, yogurt, and mango.
2. Puree the mixture until smooth.
3. Pour the entire smoothie into a bowl and decorate to make the drink look like a jack-o-lantern.
4. Use halved strawberries to make the cheeks and use the chia seeds to make eyes and a nose.
5. Serve the smoothie with a green spoon attached with a paper leaf to make it look like a pumpkin stem.

Nutrition: calories 186, fat 1, carbs 18, protein 9

Chapter 8

SALAD AND SOUPS

68. Coconut Watercress Soup

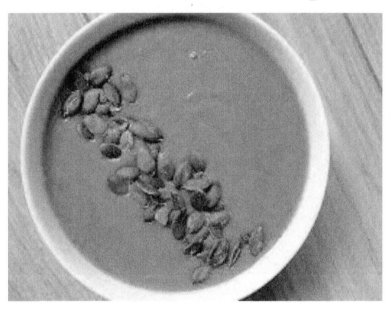

Preparation time: 10 minutes

Cooking time: 20 minutes

Servings: 4

Ingredients:

- 1 teaspoon coconut oil
- 1 onion, diced
- ¾ cup coconut milk

Directions:

1. Preparing the ingredients.
2. Melt the coconut oil in a large pot over medium-high heat. Add the onion and cook until soft, about 5 minutes, then add the peas and the water. Bring to a boil, then lower the heat and add the watercress, mint, salt, and pepper.
3. Cover and simmer for 5 minutes. Stir in the coconut milk and purée the soup until smooth in a blender or with an immersion blender.
4. Try this soup with any other fresh, leafy green—anything from spinach to collard greens to arugula to swiss chard.

Nutrition: calories 170, fat 3, carbs 18, protein 6

69. Roasted Red Pepper and Butternut Squash Soup

Preparation time: 10 minutes

Cooking time: 45 minutes

Servings: 6

Ingredients:

- 1 small butternut squash
- 1 tablespoon olive oil
- 1 teaspoon sea salt
- 2 red bell peppers
- 1 yellow onion
- 1 head garlic
- 2 cups water, or vegetable broth
- Zest and juice of 1 lime
- 1 to 2 tablespoons tahini
- Pinch cayenne pepper
- ½ teaspoon ground coriander
- ½ teaspoon ground cumin
- Toasted squash seeds (optional)

Directions:

1. Preparing the ingredients.

2. Preheat the oven to 350°f.

3. Prepare the squash for roasting by cutting it in half lengthwise, scooping out the seeds, and poking some holes in the flesh with a fork. Reserve the seeds if desired.

4. Rub a small amount of oil over the flesh and skin, then rub with a bit of sea salt and put the halves skin-side down in a large baking dish. Put it in the oven while you prepare the rest of the vegetables.

5. Prepare the peppers the exact same way, except they do not need to be poked.

6. Slice the onion in half and rub oil on the exposed faces. Slice the top off the head of garlic and rub oil on the exposed flesh.

7. After the squash has cooked for 20 minutes, add the peppers, onion, and garlic, and roast for another 20 minutes. Optionally, you can toast the squash seeds by putting them in the oven in a separate baking dish 10 to 15 minutes before the vegetables are finished.

8. Keep a close eye on them. When the vegetables are cooked, take them out and let them cool before handling them. The squash will be very soft when poked with a fork.

9. Scoop the flesh out of the squash skin into a large pot (if you have an immersion blender) or into a blender.

10. Chop the pepper roughly, remove the onion skin and chop the onion roughly, and squeeze the garlic cloves out of the head, all into the pot or blender. Add the water, the lime zest and juice, and the tahini. Purée the soup, adding more water if you like, to your desired consistency. Season with salt, cayenne, coriander, and cumin. Serve garnished with toasted squash seeds (if using).

Nutrition: calories 150, fat 3, carbs 20, protein 6

70. Tomato Pumpkin Soup

Preparation time: 25 minutes

Cooking time: 15 minutes

Servings: 4

Ingredients:

- 2 cups pumpkin, diced
- 1/2 cup tomato, chopped
- 1/2 cup onion, chopped
- 1 1/2 tsp curry powder
- 1/2 tsp paprika
- 2 cups vegetable stock
- 1 tsp olive oil
- 1/2 tsp garlic, minced

Directions:

1. In a saucepan, add oil, garlic, and onion and sauté for 3 minutes over medium heat.
2. Add remaining ingredients into the saucepan and bring to boil.
3. Reduce heat and cover and simmer for 10 minutes.
4. Puree the soup using a blender until smooth.
5. Stir well and serve warm.

Nutrition: calories 70, fat 3, carbs 13, protein 1

71. Cauliflower Spinach Soup

Preparation time: 45 minutes

Cooking time: 25 minutes

Servings: 5

Ingredients:

- 1/2 cup unsweetened coconut milk
- 5 oz fresh spinach, chopped
- 5 watercress, chopped

- 8 cups vegetable stock
- 1 lb. cauliflower, chopped
- Salt

Directions:

1. Add stock and cauliflower in a large saucepan and bring to boil over medium heat for 15 minutes.
2. Add spinach and watercress and cook for another 10 minutes.
3. Remove from heat and puree the soup using a blender until smooth.
4. Add coconut milk and stir well. Season with salt.
5. Stir well and serve hot.

Nutrition: calories 150, fat 4, carbs 8, protein 11

72. Avocado Mint Soup

Preparation time: 10 minutes

Cooking time: 10 minutes

Servings: 2

Ingredients:

- 1 medium avocado, peeled, pitted, and cut into pieces
- 1 cup coconut milk
- 2 romaine lettuce leaves
- 20 fresh mint leaves
- 1 tbsp fresh lime juice
- 1/8 tsp salt

Directions:

1. Add all ingredients into the blender and blend until smooth. The soup should be thick not as a puree.
2. Pour into the serving bowls and place in the refrigerator for 10 minutes.
3. Stir well and serve chilled.

Nutrition: calories 290, fat 3, carbs 18, protein 11

73. Creamy Squash Soup

Preparation time: 35 minutes

Cooking time: 22 minutes

Servings: 8

Ingredients:

- 3 cups butternut squash, chopped
- 1 ½ cups unsweetened coconut milk
- 1 tbsp coconut oil
- 1 tsp dried onion flakes
- 1 tbsp curry powder
- 4 cups water
- 1 garlic clove
- 1 tsp kosher salt

Directions:

1. Add squash, coconut oil, onion flakes, curry powder, water, garlic, and salt into a large saucepan. Bring to boil over high heat.
2. Turn heat to medium and simmer for 20 minutes.
3. Puree the soup using a blender until smooth. Return soup to the saucepan and stir in coconut milk and cook for 2 minutes.
4. Stir well and serve hot.

Nutrition: calories 140, fat 2, carbs 9, protein 1

74. Alkaline Carrot Soup with Fresh Mushrooms

Preparation Time: 10 minutes

Cooking Time: 20 minutes

Servings: 1-2

Ingredients:

- 4 mid-sized carrots
- 4 mid-sized potatoes
- 10 enormous new mushrooms (champignons or chanterelles)

- 1/2 white onion
- 2 tbsp. olive oil (cold squeezed, additional virgin)
- 3 cups vegetable stock
- 2 tbsp. parsley, new and cleaved
- Salt and new white pepper

Directions:

1. Wash and strip carrots and potatoes and dice them.
2. Warm-up vegetable stock in a pot on medium heat. Cook carrots and potatoes for around 15 minutes. Meanwhile finely shape onion and braise them in a container with olive oil for around 3 minutes.
3. Wash the mushrooms, slice them to the desired size, and add to the container, cooking for an additional of approximately 5 minutes, blending at times. Blend carrots, vegetable stock, and potatoes, and put the substance of the skillet into the pot.
4. When nearly done, season with parsley, salt, and pepper and serve hot. Appreciate this alkalizing soup!

Nutrition: calories 176, fat 2, carbs 23, protein 9

75. Swiss Cauliflower-Emmental-Soup

Preparation Time: 10 minutes

Cooking Time: 15 minutes

Servings: 3-4

Ingredients:

- 2 cups cauliflower pieces
- 1 cup potatoes, cubed
- 2 cups vegetable stock (without yeast)
- 3 tbsp. Swiss Emmental cheddar, cubed
- 2 tbsp. new chives
- 1 tbsp. pumpkin seeds
- 1 touch of nutmeg and cayenne pepper

Directions:

1. Cook cauliflower and potato in vegetable stock until delicate and blend it.
2. Season the soup with nutmeg and cayenne, and possibly somewhat salt and pepper.
3. Include cheddar and chives and mix a couple of moments until the soup is smooth and prepared to serve. Enhance it with pumpkin seeds.

Nutrition: calories 89, fat 1, carbs 18, protein 9

76. Chilled Parsley-Gazpacho with Lime & Cucumber

Preparation Time: 10 minutes

Cooking Time: 2 hours

Servings: 1

Ingredients:

- 4-5 middle-sized tomatoes
- 2 tbsp. olive oil, extra virgin, and cold-pressed
- 2 large cups fresh parsley
- 2 ripe avocados
- 2 cloves garlic, diced
- 2 limes, juiced
- 4 cups vegetable broth
- 1 middle-sized cucumber
- 2 small red onions, diced
- 1 tsp. dried oregano
- 1½ tsp. paprika powder
- ½ tsp. cayenne pepper
- Sea salt and freshly ground pepper to taste

Directions:

1. In a pan, heat up olive oil and sauté onions and garlic until translucent. Set aside to cool down.
2. Use a large blender and blend parsley, avocado, tomatoes, cucumber, vegetable broth, lime juice, and onion-garlic mix until smooth. Add some

water if desired, and season with cayenne pepper, paprika powder, oregano, salt, and pepper. Blend again and put in the fridge for at least 1, 5 hours.

Nutrition: calories 156, fat 1, carbs 24, protein 9

77. Chilled Avocado Tomato Soup

Preparation Time: 7 minutes

Cooking Time: 20 minutes

Servings: 1-2

Ingredients:

- 2 small avocados
- 2 large tomatoes
- 1 stalk of celery
- 1 small onion
- 1 clove of garlic
- Juice of 1 fresh lemon
- 1 cup of water (best: alkaline water)
- A handful of fresh lavages
- Parsley and sea salt to taste

Directions:

1. Scoop the avocados and cut all veggies into little pieces.
2. Spot all fixings in a blender and blend until smooth.
3. Serve chilled and appreciate this nutritious and sound soluble soup formula!

Nutrition: calories 210, fat 1, carbs 18, protein 9

78. Pumpkin and White Bean Soup with Sage

Preparation Time: 10 minutes

Cooking Time: 40 minutes

Servings: 3-4

Ingredients:

- 1 ½ pound pumpkin
- ½ pound yams
- ½ pound white beans
- 1 onion
- 2 cloves of garlic
- 1 tbsp. of cold squeezed additional virgin olive oil
- 1 tbsp. of spices (your top picks)
- 1 tbsp. of sage
- 1 ½ quart water (best: antacid water)
- A spot of ocean salt and pepper

Directions:

1. Cut the pumpkin and potatoes in shapes, cut the onion, and cut the garlic, the spices, and the sage in fine pieces.
2. Sauté the onion and also the garlic in olive oil for around two or three minutes.
3. Include the potatoes, pumpkin, spices, and sage and fry for an additional 5 minutes.
4. At that point include the water and cook for around 30 minutes (spread the pot with a top) until vegetables are delicate.
5. At long last include the beans and some salt and pepper. Cook for an additional 5 minutes and serve right away. Prepared!! Appreciate this antacid soup. Alkalizing tasty!

Nutrition: calories 218, fat 1, carbs 11, protein 8

79. Alkaline Carrot Soup with Millet

Preparation Time: 7 minutes

Cooking Time: 40 minutes

Servings: 3-4

Ingredients:

- 2 cups cauliflower pieces
- 1 cup potatoes, cubed

- 2 cups vegetable stock (without yeast)
- 3 tbsp. Swiss Emmental cheddar, cubed
- 2 tbsp. new chives
- 1 tbsp. pumpkin seeds
- 1 touch of nutmeg and cayenne pepper

Directions:

1. Cook cauliflower and potato in vegetable stock until delicate and blend it.
2. Season the soup with nutmeg and cayenne, and possibly somewhat salt and pepper.
3. Include Emmental cheddar and chives and mix a couple of moments until the soup is smooth and prepared to serve. It can be enhanced with pumpkin seeds.

Nutrition: calories 90, fat 1, carbs 18, protein 11

80. Alkaline Pumpkin Tomato Soup

Preparation Time: 15 minutes

Cooking Time: 30 minutes

Servings: 3-4

Ingredients:

- 1 quart of water (if accessible: soluble water)
- 400g new tomatoes, stripped and diced
- 1 medium-sized sweet pumpkin
- 5 yellow onions
- 1 tbsp. cold squeezed additional virgin olive oil
- 2 tsp. ocean salt or natural salt
- Touch of cayenne pepper
- Your preferred spices (discretionary)
- Bunch of new parsley

Directions:

1. Cut onions in little pieces and sauté with some oil in a significant pot.
2. Cut the pumpkin down the middle, at that point remove the stem and scoop out the seeds.
3. At long last scoop out the fragile living creature and put it in the pot.
4. Include likewise the tomatoes and the water and cook for around 20 minutes.
5. At that point empty the soup into a food processor and blend well for a couple of moments. Sprinkle with salt, pepper, and other spices.
6. Fill bowls and trimming with new parsley. Make the most of your alkalizing soup!

Nutrition: calories 190, fat 3, carbs 18, protein 11

81. Alkaline Pumpkin Coconut Soup

Preparation Time: 10 minutes

Cooking Time: 15 minutes

Servings: 3-4

Ingredients:

- 2 lb pumpkin
- 6 cups of water (best: soluble water delivered with a water ionizer)
- 1 cup low-fat coconut milk
- 5 ounces of potatoes
- 2 major onions
- 3 ounces leek
- 1 bunch of new parsley
- 1 touch of nutmeg
- 1 touch of cayenne pepper
- 1 tsp. ocean salt or natural salt
- 4 tbsp. cold squeezed additional virgin olive oil

Directions:

1. As a matter of first significance: cut the onions, the pumpkin, and the potatoes just as the hole into little pieces.

2. At that point, heat the olive oil in a significant pot and sauté the onions for a couple of moments.

3. At that point, include the water and heat up the pumpkin, potatoes, and the leek until delicate.

4. Include coconut milk.

5. Presently utilize a hand blender and puree for around 1 moment. The soup should turn out to be extremely velvety.

6. Season with salt, pepper, and nutmeg. Lastly, include the parsley and appreciate this alkalizing pumpkin soup hot or cold!

Nutrition: calories 90, fat 3, carbs 23, protein 1

82. Cold Cauliflower-Coconut Soup

Preparation Time: 7 minutes

Cooking Time: 20 minutes

Servings: 3-4

Ingredients:

- 1 pound (450g) new cauliflower
- 1 ¼ cup (300ml) unsweetened coconut milk
- 1 cup of water (best: antacid water)
- 2 tbsp. new lime juice
- 1/3 cup cold squeezed additional virgin olive oil
- 1 cup new coriander leaves, slashed
- Spot of salt and cayenne pepper
- 1 bunch of unsweetened coconut chips

Directions:

1. Steam cauliflower for around 10 minutes.

2. At that point, set up the cauliflower with coconut milk and water in a food processor and get it started until extremely smooth.

3. Include new lime squeeze, salt and pepper, a large portion of the cleaved coriander, and the oil and blend for an additional couple of moments.

4. Pour in soup bowls and embellishment with coriander and coconut chips. Enjoy!

Nutrition: calories 190, fat 1, carbs 21, protein 6

83. Raw Avocado-Broccoli Soup with Cashew Nuts

Preparation Time: 10 minutes

Cooking Time: 30 minutes

Servings: 1-2

Ingredients:

- ½ cup of water (if available: alkaline water)
- ½ avocado
- 1 cup chopped broccoli
- ½ cup cashew nuts
- ½ cup alfalfa sprouts
- 1 clove of garlic
- 1 tbsp. cold-pressed extra virgin olive oil
- 1 pinch of sea salt and pepper
- Some parsley to garnish

Directions:

1. Put the cashew nuts in a blender or food processor, include some water and puree for a couple of moments.
2. Include the various fixings (except for the avocado) individually and puree each an ideal opportunity for a couple of moments.
3. Dispense the soup in a container and warm it up to the normal room temperature. Enhance with salt and pepper. In the interim dice the avocado and slash the parsley.
4. Dispense the soup in a container or plate; include the avocado slices and embellishment with parsley.
5. That's it! Enjoy this excellent healthy soup!

Nutrition: calories 48, fat 1, carbs 21, protein 8

84. Chilled Cucumber and Lime Soup

Preparation Time: 5 minutes

Cooking Time: 20 minutes

Servings: 1-2

Chilled soups are perfect for the hot summer months, and this easy soup is made with garden fresh vegetables with no cooking involved. Simply prepare the veggies, add them to a blender, and lunch is served!

Ingredients:

- 1 cucumber, peeled
- ½ zucchini, peeled
- 1 tablespoon freshly squeezed lime juice
- 1 tablespoon fresh cilantro leaves
- 1 garlic clove, crushed
- ¼ teaspoon of sea salt

Directions:

1. In a blender, blend the cucumber, zucchini, lime juice, cilantro, garlic, and salt until well combined. Add more salt, if necessary.
2. Fill 1 huge or 2 little dishes and enjoy immediately or refrigerate for 15 to 20 minutes to chill before serving.

Nutrition: calories 90, fat 1, carbs 12, protein 5

85. Lime & Mint Summer Fruit Salad

Preparation Time: 10 minutes

Cooking Time: 0 minutes

Serving: 4

Ingredients:

- ¼ cup apple, peeled and diced
- ¼ cup grapes
- 2 tablespoons mint, fresh and chopped
- 2 tablespoons Seville orange juice, freshly squeezed

- ¼ cup strawberries
- ¼ cup peaches, peeled and diced
- ¼ cup tangerine slices
- ¼ cup cantaloupe, small bite-size pieces
- ¼ cup honeydew melon, small bite-size pieces
- ¼ cup watermelon, small bite-size pieces

Directions:

1. In a mixing bowl, combine all of the fruit.
2. Add the Seville orange juice, mint, and mix well.
3. Serve chilled and enjoy!

Nutrition: calories 185, fat 1, carbs 18, protein 1

86. Cherry Tomato & Kale Salad

Preparation Time: 10 minutes

Cooking Time: 0 minutes

Serving: 2

Ingredients:

- 2 tbsps. Ranch dressing
- 2 cups organic baby tomatoes
- 1 bunch kale, stemmed, leaves washed and chopped

Directions:

1. Mix all the ingredients in a bowl.
2. Divide the salad equally into two serving dishes.
3. Serve.

Nutrition: calories 116, fat 1, carbs 12, protein 8

87. Radish Noodle Salad

Preparation Time: 10 minutes

Cooking Time: 0 minutes

Serving: 4

Ingredients:

- 2 cups cooked radish florets
- 1 roasted spaghetti squash
- 1 chopped scallion
- 1 tbsp. sesame oil
- 1 bell seeded pepper, cut into strips
- 2 tbsps. Toasted sesame seeds
- 1 tsp. sea salt
- 1 tsp. red pepper flakes

Directions:

1. Start by preparing the spaghetti squash by removing the cooked squash with a fork into a bowl.
2. Add the radish, red bell pepper, and scallion to the bowl with the squash.
3. In a small bowl, mix the red pepper flakes, salt, and sesame oil.
4. Drizzle the mixture to top the vegetables. Toss gently to combine them.
5. Add the sesame seeds to garnish.
6. Serve.

Nutrition: calories 112, fat 1, carbs 8, protein 2

88. Caprese Salad

Preparation Time: 5 minutes

Cooking Time: 0 minutes

Serving: 2

Ingredients:

- 1 sliced avocado
- 2 sliced large tomatoes
- 1 bunch basil leaves
- 1 tsp. sea salt
- 1 cup cubed jackfruit

Directions:

1. In a bowl toss all the salad ingredients to mix.
2. Add the sea salt to season.
3. Serve.

Nutrition: calories 125, fat 1, carbs 18, protein 3

89. Summer Lettuce Salad

Preparation Time: 5 minutes

Cooking Time: 0 minutes

Serving: 4

Ingredients:

- 2 cups halved cherry tomatoes
- 4 cups romaine lettuce or iceberg
- 1 peeled and sliced cucumber
- 2 thinly sliced radishes
- 1 sliced scallion
- 1/2 cup shredded zucchini
- 14 oz. can drained whole green beans

Directions:

1. Add all of the salad ingredients in a large bowl then toss with 2 tbsps. Of the dressing.
2. Serve.

Nutrition: calories 143, fat 1, carbs 12, protein 1

90. Mustard Cabbage Salad

Preparation Time: 10 Minutes

Cooking Time: 0

Servings: 4

Ingredients:

- 1 green cabbage head, shredded
- 1 red cabbage head, shredded
- 2 tablespoons avocado oil
- 2 tablespoons mustard
- 1 tablespoon balsamic vinegar
- 1 teaspoon hot paprika
- Salt and black pepper to the taste
- 1 tablespoon dill, chopped

Directions:

1. In a bowl, mix the cabbage with the oil, mustard, and the other ingredients, toss, divide between plates and serve as a side salad.

Nutrition: calories 150, fat 1, carbs 6, protein 3

91. Alkaline-Electric Spring Salad

Preparation Time: 11 minutes

Cooking Time: 15 Minutes

Serving: 2

Ingredients

- 1 cup cherry tomatoes
- 4 cups seasonal greens
- 1/4 cup walnuts
- 1/4 cup approved herbs
- For the dressing:
- Sea salt and cayenne pepper
- 3 key limes
- 1 tablespoon of homemade raw sesame tahini butter

Directions:

1. Sap the key limes.
2. Whisk together the homemade raw sesame "tahini" butter with the key lime juice in a small bowl.

3. Add cayenne pepper and sea salt to your satisfaction.
4. Cut the cherry tomatoes in half.
5. In a large bowl, combine the greens, cherry tomatoes, and herbs. Pour the dressing on top and massage with your hands.
6. Let the greens soak the dressing. Add more cayenne pepper, herbs, and sea salt.
7. Enjoy

Nutrition: calories 218, fat 1, carbs 19, protein 2

92. Super Healthy Beet Greens Salad

Preparation Time: 10 Minutes

Cooking Time: 0

Servings: 4

Ingredients:

For Dressing:

- 1 garlic clove, minced
- 1 ½ teaspoons of Dijon mustard
- 3 tablespoons of extra-virgin olive oil
- 1 tablespoon balsamic vinegar
- Salt and freshly ground black pepper, to taste
- 2 cups of vegetable broth
- ¼ cup of olive oil

For Salad:

- 8 cup of fresh beet greens
- ¼ cup of feta cheese, crumbled

Directions:

1. Prepare dressing in a bowl by adding all the dressing ingredients and beat until well combined.
2. In a large bowl, mix together greens and cheese.
3. Pour dressing over salad and toss to coat well. Serve immediately.

Nutrition: calories 250, fat 1, carbs 19, protein 1

93. Super Delicious Cucumber Salad

Preparation Time: 10 Minutes

Cooking Time: 0

Servings: 8

Ingredients:

- ½ cup of sour cream
- 1 teaspoon of white vinegar
- ½ teaspoon of powdered stevia
- ½ teaspoon of dill weed
- Salt, to taste
- 4 medium cucumbers, sliced

Directions:

1. In a bowl, add all the ingredients except cucumbers and beat until well combined.
2. Add cucumber slices and stir until well combined.
3. Refrigerate to chill for at least 30 minutes before serving.

Nutrition: calories 84, fat 1, carbs 10, protein 1

94. Nutty and Fruity Garden Salad

Preparation time: 10 minutes

Cooking time: 0 minutes

Servings: 2

Ingredients:

- 6 cups baby spinach
- ½ cup chopped walnuts, toasted
- 1 ripe red pear, sliced
- 1 ripe persimmon, sliced
- 1 teaspoon garlic minced
- 1 shallot, minced
- 1 tablespoon extra-virgin olive oil

- 2 tablespoons fresh lemon juice
- 1 teaspoon wholegrain mustard

Directions:

1. Mix well garlic, shallot, oil, lemon juice, and mustard in a large salad bowl.
2. Add spinach, pear, and persimmon. Toss to coat well.
3. To serve, garnish with chopped pecans.

Nutrition: calories 330, fat 1, carbs 18, protein 1

95. A Snowy "Frozen" Salad Bowl

Preparation Time: 75 Minutes

Cooking Time: 0

Servings: 3

Ingredients:

- ½ a cup of white sugar
- 2 cups of water
- 1 can of 20-ounce frozen orange juice concentrate (thawed)
- 1 can of 20-ounce frozen lemonade concentrated (thawed)
- 4 bananas, sliced
- 1 can have crushed pineapple (with juice)
- 1 pack of strawberries (thawed)

Directions:

1. Take a bowl and add water and sugar
2. Dissolve the sugar and add orange juice, bananas, lemonade, crushed pineapples (alongside the juice), and strawberries and give it a nice mix
3. Pour the mixture into a 9x13 inch glass pan and allow it to chill
4. Once ready to serve, let it sit for about 5 minutes at room temp and cut them out

Nutrition: calories 210, fat 1, carbs 21, protein 1

96. Warm Mushroom and Orange Pepper Salad

Preparation Time: 10 Minutes

Cooking Time: 8 Minutes

Servings: 4

Ingredients:

- 2 tbsp. avocado oil
- 1 cup mixed mushrooms, chopped
- 2 orange bell peppers, deseeded and finely sliced
- 1 garlic clove, minced
- 2 tbsp. tamarind sauce
- 1 tsp. maple (sugar-free) syrup
- ½ tsp. hot sauce
- ½ tsp. fresh ginger paste
- Sesame seeds to garnish

Directions:

1. Over medium fire, heat half of avocado oil in a large skillet, sauté mushroom, and bell peppers until slightly softened, 5 minutes.
2. In a small bowl, whisk garlic, tamarind sauce, maple syrup, hot sauce, and ginger paste. Add mixture to vegetables and stir-fry for 2 to 3 minutes.
3. Turn heat off and dish salad. Drizzle with remaining avocado oil and garnish with sesame seeds.
4. Serve with grilled tofu.

Nutrition: calories 290, fat 1, carbs 8, protein 1

97. Broccoli, Kelp, and Feta Salad

Preparation Time: 15 Minutes

Cooking Time: 0

Servings: 4

Ingredients:

- 2 tbsp. olive oil
- 1 tbsp. white wine vinegar
- 2 tbsp. chia seeds
- Salt and freshly ground black pepper to taste
- 2 cups broccoli slaw
- 1 cup chopped kelp, thoroughly washed, and steamed
- 1/3 cup chopped pecans
- 1/3 cup pumpkin seeds
- 1/3 cup blueberries
- 2/3 cup ricotta cheese

Directions:

1. In a small bowl, whisk olive oil, white wine vinegar, chia seeds, salt, and black pepper. Set aside.
2. In a large salad bowl, combine the broccoli slaw, kelp, pecans, pumpkin seeds, blueberries, and ricotta cheese.
3. Drizzle dressing on top, toss, and serve.

Nutrition: calories 390, fat 3, carbs 8, protein 8

98. Roasted Asparagus with Feta Cheese Salad

Preparation Time: 10 minutes

Cooking Time: 20 minutes

Serving: 4

Ingredients:

- 1 lb. asparagus, trimmed and halved
- 2 tbsp. olive oil
- ½ tsp. dried basil
- ½ tsp. dried oregano
- Salt and freshly ground black pepper to taste
- ½ tsp. hemp seeds
- 1 tbsp. maple (sugar-free) syrup

- ½ cup arugula
- 4 tbsp. crumbled feta cheese
- 2 tbsp. hazelnuts
- 1 lemon, cut into wedges

Directions:

1. Preheat oven to 3500F.
2. Pour asparagus on a baking tray, drizzle with olive oil, basil, oregano, salt, black pepper, and hemp seeds. Mix with your hands and roast in the oven for 15 minutes.
3. Remove, drizzle with maple syrup, and continue cooking until slightly charred for 5 minutes.
4. Spread arugula in a salad bowl and top with asparagus. Scatter with feta cheese, hazelnuts, and serve with lemon wedges.

Nutrition: calories 140, fat 3, carbs 18, protein 4

99. Fresh Veggie Salad

Preparation Time: 20 Minutes

Cooking Time: 0

Servings: 8

Ingredients:

For Dressing:

- 5 tablespoons olive oil
- 3 tablespoons fresh lemon juice
- 2 tablespoons fresh mint leaves, chopped finely
- 1 teaspoon Erythritol
- Salt and freshly ground black pepper, to taste

For Salad:

- 2 cups cucumbers, peeled and sliced
- 2 cups tomatoes, sliced
- 1 cup black olives
- 6 cups lettuce

- 1 cup mozzarella cheese, cubed

Directions:

1. For the dressing: in a bowl, add all ingredients and beat until well combined.
2. Cover and refrigerate to chill for about 1 hour.
3. For the salad: in a large serving bowl, add all ingredients and mix.
4. Pour dressing over salad and toss to coat well.
5. Serve immediately.

Nutrition: calories 321, fat 1, carbs 8, protein 1

100. Strawberry Salad

Preparation Time: 15 Minutes

Cooking Time: 0

Servings: 4

Ingredients:

- 6 cups fresh baby greens
- 2 cups fresh strawberries, hulled and sliced
- 1 tablespoon fresh mint leaves
- ¼ cup olive oil
- 2 tablespoons fresh lemon juice
- ¼ teaspoon liquid stevia
- 1/8 teaspoon paprika
- 1/8 teaspoon garlic powder
- Salt, to taste

Directions:

1. For the salad: in a large serving bowl, add greens, strawberries, and mint and mix.
2. For the dressing: in a bowl, add remaining ingredients and beat until well combined.
3. Pour dressing over salad and toss to coat well.
4. Serve immediately.

Nutrition: calories 141, fat 2, carbs 18, protein 9

101. Tex Mex Black Bean and Avocado Salad

Preparation Time: 15 Minutes

Cooking Time: 0

Servings: 2

Ingredients:

- 14 oz. black beans, drained and rinsed
- 3 jars roasted red peppers, chopped
- 1 avocado, chopped
- ½ onion, chopped
- 1 red chili, chopped
- 1 lime, plus wedges to serve
- Olive oil
- 1 teaspoon cumin seeds
- 2 handfuls rocket
- 2 pitta breads, warmed

Directions:

1. Combine beans, peppers, avocado, onion, and chili in a large mixing bowl.
2. Add lime juice, cumin seeds, and mix well.
3. Serve the rocket on two plates with warm pittas and divide the bean mixture.

Nutrition: calories 120, fat 3, carbs 8, protein 5

102. Sweet Potato Salad

Preparation: 10 Minutes

Cooking Time: 30 Minutes

Servings: 4

Ingredients:

- 2 sweet potatoes, peeled and cubed
- 1 tablespoon olive oil
- ½ teaspoon each of paprika, oregano, and cayenne pepper
- 1 shallot, diced

- 2 spring onions, chopped
- 1 small bunch chives, chopped
- 3 tablespoons red wine vinegar
- 2 teaspoons olive oil
- 1 tablespoon pure maple syrup
- Salt and pepper

Directions:

1. Preheat the oven to 300F and prepare a baking sheet by lining it with parchment paper.
2. Place sweet potatoes on the baking sheet.
3. Drizzle some olive oil and spices, toss well, and bake for 30 minutes.
4. In a separate bowl, mix shallots, scallions, chives, vinegar, olive oil, and maple syrup.
5. Add baked sweet potatoes to the dressing.

Nutrition: calories 169, fat 1, carbs 5, protein 1

103. Lentil Salad with Spinach and Pomegranate

Preparation Time: 15 Minutes

Cooking Time: 0

Servings: 3

Ingredients

For the vegan lentil salad:

- 3 cups brown lentils, cooked
- 1 avocado, cut into slices
- 2-3 handfuls fresh spinach
- ½ cup walnuts, chopped
- 2 apples, chopped
- 1 pomegranate

For the tahini orange dressing:

- 3 tablespoons tahini
- 2 tablespoons olive oil

- 1 clove of garlic
- 6 tablespoons water
- 4 tablespoons orange juice
- 2 teaspoons orange zest
- Salt and pepper

Directions:

1. Prepare lentils according to package instructions.
2. Place pomegranate in a shallow bowl filled with water, cut in half, and take out seeds, remove fibers floating on the water.
3. Process all dressing ingredients in a food processor. Process until smooth and set aside.
4. Place salad ingredients in a large bowl and mix well.
5. Drizzle dressing over salad before serving.

Nutrition: calories 104, fat 3, carbs 18, protein 11

104. Broccoli Salad Curry Dressing

Preparation Time: 30 Minutes

Cooking Time: 0

Servings: 6

Ingredients:

- ½ cup plain, unsweetened vegan yogurt
- ¼ cup onion, chopped
- 2 heads broccoli florets, chopped
- 2 stalks celery, chopped
- ½ teaspoon curry powder
- ¼ teaspoon salt or to taste
- 2 tablespoons sunflower seeds

Directions:

1. Mix yogurt, curry powder, and salt.
2. Toss broccoli florets, celery onion, and sunflower seeds.
3. Drizzle the dressing on top and put the salad in the fridge for 30 minutes.

Nutrition: calories 167, fat 1, carbs 18, protein 1

105. Cherry Tomato Salad with Soy Chorizo

Preparation Time: 5 Minutes

Cooking Time: 5 Minutes

Servings: 4

Ingredients:

- 2 ½ tbsp. olive oil
- 4 soy chorizos, chopped
- 2 tsp. red wine vinegar
- 1 small red onion, finely chopped
- 2 ½ cups cherry tomatoes, halved
- 2 tbsp. chopped cilantro
- Salt and freshly ground black pepper to taste
- 3 tbsp. sliced black olives to garnish

Directions:

1. Heat half a tablespoon of olive oil in a skillet over a medium heat and fry soy chorizo until golden. Turn heat off.
2. In a salad bowl, whisk remaining olive oil and vinegar. Add onion, cilantro, tomatoes, and soy chorizo. Mix with dressing and season with salt and black pepper.
3. Garnish with olives and serve.

Nutrition: calories 130, fat 1, carbs 7, protein 1

106. Roasted Bell Pepper Salad with Olives

Preparation Time: 10 Minutes

Cooking Time: 20 Minutes

Servings: 4

Ingredients:

- 8 large red bell peppers, deseeded and cut in wedges
- ½ tsp. erythritol

- 2 ½ tbsp. olive oil
- 1/3 cup arugula
- 1 tbsp. mint leaves
- 1/3 cup pitted Kalamata olives
- 3 tbsp. chopped almonds
- ½ tbsp. balsamic vinegar
- Crumbled feta cheese for topping
- Toasted pine nuts for topping

Directions:

1. Preheat oven to 400 F.
2. Pour bell peppers on a roasting pan; season with erythritol and drizzle with half of the olive oil. Roast in oven until slightly charred, 20 minutes. Remove from the oven and set aside.
3. Arrange arugula in a salad bowl, scatter bell peppers on top, mint leaves, olives, almonds, and drizzle with balsamic vinegar and remaining olive oil. Season with salt and black pepper.
4. Toss, top with feta cheese and pine nuts, and serve.

Nutrition: calories 145, fat 1, carbs 8, protein 1

107. Tofu-Dulse-Walnut Salad

Preparation Time: 10 Minutes

Cooking Time: 15 Minutes

Servings: 4

Ingredients:

- 1 (7 oz.) block extra firm tofu
- 2 tbsp. olive oil
- 2 tbsp. butter
- 1 cup asparagus, trimmed and halved
- 1 cup green beans, trimmed
- 2 tbsp. chopped dulse
- Salt and freshly ground black pepper to taste
- ½ lemon, juiced

- 4 tbsp. chopped walnuts

Directions:

1. Place tofu in between two paper towels and allow soaking for 5 minutes. After, remove towels and chop into small cubes.
2. Heat olive oil in a skillet and fry tofu until golden, 10 minutes. Remove onto a paper towel-lined plate and set aside.
3. Melt butter in a skillet and sauté asparagus and green beans until softened, 5 minutes. Add dulse, season with salt and black pepper, and cook until softened. Mix in tofu and stir-fry for 5 minutes.
4. Plate, drizzle with lemon juice, and scatter walnuts on top.
5. Serve warm.

Nutrition: calories 178, fat 1, carbs 9, protein 1

108. Green Quinoa Salad

Preparation Time: 5 minutes

Cooking Time: 0 minutes

Serving: 4

Ingredients:

- 1 cup trimmed, cooked, and roughly chopped asparagus spears
- 1 cup roughly chopped radish florets
- 1/2 tsp. sea salt
- 2 tbsps. Coconut oil
- 2 tbsps. Freshly squeezed Seville orange juice
- 1/2 cup water
- 2 cups cooled cooked quinoa

Directions:

1. In a bowl, mix the radish and asparagus.
2. Add in the quinoa then stir.
3. Mix the water, coconut oil, salt, and Seville orange juice using a blender.
4. Blend until the ingredients emulsify.
5. Pour the mixture over the salad then stir to mix.
6. Keep the salad in the fridge for about 15 minutes to chill.

7. Serve cold.

Nutrition: calories 121, fat 1, carbs 11, protein 1

109. Salad Pop

Preparation Time: 5 minutes

Cooking Time: 0 minutes

Serving: 4

Ingredients:

- 1 yellow squash, sliced into pieces
- 1 zucchini, sliced into pieces
- 1 cucumber, sliced into pieces
- 8 cauliflower florets
- 2 tbsps. Blue cheese dressing
- 8 steamed radish florets
- 8 cherry tomatoes

Directions:

1. Thread 1 zucchini slice onto a wooden skewer, followed by the 1 yellow squash slice, 1 cucumber, 1 cherry tomato, 1 radish floret, and 1 cauliflower floret.
2. Repeat the process with the remaining ingredients and vegetable pieces.
3. Drizzle with the blue cheese dressing.
4. Serve.

Nutrition: calories 143, fat 1, carbs 18, protein 7

110. Avocado Power Salad

Preparation Time: 10 minutes

Cooking Time: 0 minutes

Serving: 2

Ingredients:

- 1 cubed avocado
- 1 cup cooled cooked quinoa
- 1 tbsp. freshly squeezed Seville orange juice
- 1 tsp. sea salt
- 1 tbsp. onion powder
- 1 tbsp. onion powder
- 1/4 cup chopped cilantro
- 1 cup peeled and diced cucumber
- 1 cup halved cherry tomatoes
- 5oz. fresh and roughly chopped kale

Directions:

1. Mix all the ingredients.
2. Place the mixture in the fridge to chill for about 15 minutes
3. Serve.

Nutrition: calories 211, fat 2, carbs 18, protein 5

111. Wakame Salad

Preparation Time: 10 minutes

Cooking Time: 15 minutes

Serving: 2

Ingredients

- 2 cups of Wakame Stems
- 1 tablespoon of Sesame Seeds
- 2 tablespoons of diced Red Bell Pepper
- 1 teaspoon of Ginger
- 1 tablespoon of Agave Syrup
- 1 teaspoon of Onion Powder
- 1 tablespoon of Sesame Oil
- 1 tablespoon of Key Lime juice
- Spring Water for soaking

Direction:

1. Put wakame stems in a medium bowl and cover them with spring water.
2. Soak wakame stems for 8 to 10 minutes until soft then drain the water.
3. In a separate bowl, combine agave syrup, onion powder, sesame oil, ginger, and key lime juice and whisk them thoroughly.
4. Place diced bell pepper and soaked wakame on a plate. Pour dressing over the salad.
5. Sprinkle sesame seeds on top.
6. Enjoy your wakame salad!

Nutrition: calories 190, fat 1, carbs 18, protein 1

112. Healthy Salad

Preparation Time: 10 minutes

Cooking Time: 54 minutes

Serving: 2

Ingredients

- 2 cups of torn Watercress
- 1/2 of sliced Cucumber
- 1 tablespoon of Key Lime Juice
- 2 tablespoons of Olive Oil
- Pure Sea Salt, to taste
- Cayenne Powder, to taste

Direction:

1. Pour key lime juice and olive oil into a salad bowl. Mix them well to combine.
2. Slice the cucumber and add to the bowl.
3. Tear watercress and add to the bowl.
4. Sprinkle cayenne powder and pure sea salt on top according to your liking.
5. Mix thoroughly.
6. Enjoy your quick detox salad!

Nutrition: calories 265, fat 1, carbs 9, protein 1

Chapter 9

SPECIAL INGREDIENTS

113. Homemade Hemp Seed Milk

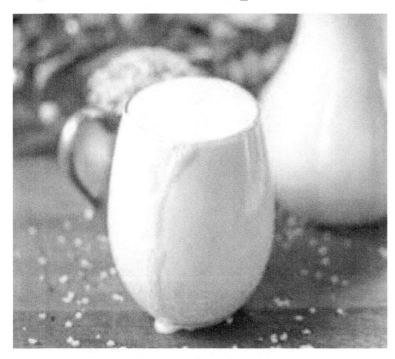

Preparation Time: 15 minutes

Cooking Time: 2 hours

Servings: 2

Ingredients:

- 2 tablespoons of hemp seeds
- 2 tablespoons of agave syrup

- 1/8 teaspoon of pure sea salt
- 2 cups of spring water
- Fruits (optional)*

Directions:

1. Place all ingredients, except fruits, into the blender.
2. Blend them for two minutes.
3. Add fruits and repeatedly blend for 30 to 50 seconds.
4. Leave milk in a refrigerator until cold.
5. Enjoy your homemade hemp seed milk!

Nutrition: calories 211, fat 1, carbs 8, protein 1

114. Italian Infused Oil

Preparation Time: 5 minutes

Cooking Time: 24 hours

Servings: 1

Ingredients:

- 1 teaspoon of oregano
- 1 teaspoon of basil
- 1 pinch of pure sea salt
- 3/4 cup of grapeseed oil

Directions:

1. Fill a glass jar with a lid or a squeeze bottle with grapeseed oil.
2. Mix seasoning together and add them to the jar/bottle.
3. Shake it and let the oil infuse for at least 24 hours.
4. Add it to a dish and enjoy your Italian infused oil!

Nutrition: calories 120, fat 1, carbs 10, protein 1

115. Garlic Infused Oil

Preparation Time: 5 minutes

Cooking Time: 24 hours

Servings: 1

Ingredients:

- 1/2 teaspoon of dill
- 1/2 teaspoon of ginger powder
- 1 tablespoon of onion powder
- 1/2 teaspoon of pure sea salt
- 3/4 cup of grapeseed oil

Directions:

1. Fill a glass jar with a lid or a squeeze bottle with Grape Seed Oil.
2. Add the seasonings to the jar/bottle.
3. Shake it and let the oil infuse for at least 24 hours.
4. Add it to a dish and enjoy your "Garlic" Infused Oil!

Nutrition: calories 130, fat 4, carbs 19, protein 2

116. Papaya Seed Mango Dressing

Preparation Time: 5 minutes

Cooking Time: 10 minutes

Servings: 2

Ingredients:

- 1 cup of chopped mango
- 1 teaspoon of ground papaya seeds
- 1 teaspoon of basil
- 1 teaspoon of onion powder
- 1 teaspoon of agave syrup
- 2 tablespoons of lime juice
- 1/4 cup of grapeseed oil
- 1/4 teaspoon of pure sea salt

Directions:

1. Prepare and place all ingredients into the blender.
2. Blend for one minute until smooth.
3. Add it to a salad and enjoy your papaya seed mango dressing!

Nutrition: calories 320, fat 12, carbs 18, protein 1

117. Tomato Ginger Dressing

Preparation Time: 5 minutes

Cooking Time: 10 minutes

Servings: 2

Ingredients:

- 2 chopped plum tomatoes
- 1 teaspoon of minced ginger*
- 1 tablespoon of agave syrup
- 2 tablespoons of chopped onion
- 2 tablespoons of sesame seeds
- 1 tablespoon of lime juice

Directions:

1. Prepare and place all ingredients into the blender.
2. Blend for one minute until smooth.
3. Add it to a salad and enjoy your tomato ginger dressing!

Nutrition: calories 1, fat 3, carbs 18, protein 11

118. Dill Cucumber Dressing

Preparation Time: 5 minutes

Cooking Time: 10 minutes

Servings: 2

Ingredients:

- 1 teaspoon of fresh dill*
- 1 cup of quartered cucumbers
- 1/2 teaspoon of onion powder
- 2 teaspoons of agave syrup
- 1 tablespoon of lime juice
- 1/4 cup of Avocado oil

Directions:

1. Prepare and place all ingredients into the blender.
2. Blend for one minute until smooth.
3. Add it to a salad and enjoy your dill cucumber dressing!

Nutrition: calories 111, fat 3, carbs 18, protein 11

119. Homemade Walnut Milk

Preparation Time: 15 minutes

Cooking Time: Minimum 8 hours

Servings: 4 cups

Ingredients:

- 1 cup of raw walnuts
- 1/8 teaspoon of pure sea salt
- 3 cups of spring water + extra for soaking

Directions:

1. Put raw walnuts in a small pot and cover them with three inches of water.
2. Soak the walnuts for at least eight hours.
3. Drain and rinse the walnuts with cold water.
4. Add the soaked walnuts, pure sea salt, and three cups of spring water to a blender.
5. Mix well until smooth.
6. Strain it if you need to.
7. Enjoy your homemade walnut milk!

Nutrition: calories 118, fat 111, carbs 18, protein 1

120. Aquafaba

Preparation Time: 15 minutes

Cooking Time: 2 Hours 30 Minutes

Servings: 2-4 Cups

Ingredients:

- 1 bag of garbanzo beans
- 1 teaspoon of pure sea salt
- 6 cups of spring water + extra for soaking

Directions:

1. Place garbanzo beans in a large pot, add spring water and pure sea salt. Bring to a rolling boil.
2. Remove from the heat and leave to soak kindly for 30 to 40 minutes.
3. Strain garbanzo beans and add 6 cups of spring water.
4. Boil for 1 hour and 30 minutes on medium heat.
5. Strain the garbanzo beans. This strained water is Aquafaba.
6. Pour Aquafaba into a glass jar with a lid and place it into the refrigerator.
7. After cooling, Aquafaba becomes thicker. If it is too liquid, repeatedly boil for 10-20 minutes.

Nutrition: calories 234, fat 10, carbs 9, protein 11

121. Potato and Zucchini Casserole

Preparation Time: 10 Minutes

Cooking Time: 1 hour

Servings: 6

Ingredients:

- ¾ cup nutritional yeast
- ¾ cup diced green or red bell pepper (about one small bell pepper)
- ¾ cup diced red, white, or yellow onion (about one small onion)
- ½ cup dry breadcrumbs
- ¼ cup olive oil (optional)
- 1½ teaspoons minced garlic (about three small cloves)
- Pepper, to taste
- Sea salt, to taste (optional)

Directions:

1. Preheat the oven to 400°F.
2. Mix all the ingredients.
3. Place the mixture in a large cooking pot dish.
4. Bake in a preheated oven for 1 hour until heated through, stirring once halfway through.
5. Take off from the oven and allow to cool for 5 minutes before serving.

Nutrition: calories 321, fat 10, carbs 38, protein 14

122. Broccoli Casserole with Beans and Walnuts

Preparation Time: 10 Minutes

Cooking Time: 35-40 Minutes

Servings: 4

Ingredients:

- ¾ cup vegetable broth
- Two broccoli heads, crowns, and stalks finely chopped
- One teaspoon salt (optional)
- 2 cups cooked pinto or navy beans
- 1 to 2 tablespoons brown rice flour or arrowroot flour
- 1 cup chopped walnuts

Directions:

1. Preheat the oven to 400°F (205°C).
2. Warm the vegetable broth in a large ovenproof pot over medium heat.
3. Add the broccoli and season with salt, if desired, then cook for 6 to 8 minutes, stirring occasionally, or until the broccoli is light green.
4. Add the pinto beans and brown rice flour to the skillet and stir well. Sauté for another 5 to 7 minutes, or until the liquid thickens slightly. Scatter the top with the walnuts.
5. Transfer the pot to the oven. Bake it until the walnuts are toasted, 20 to 25 minutes.
6. Let the casserole cool for 8 to 10 minutes in the pot before serving.

Nutrition: calories 419, fat 2, carbs 18, protein 11

123. Pistachio Crusted Tofu

Preparation Time: 10 Minutes

Cooking Time: 20 Minutes

Servings: 8

Ingredients:

- ½ cup roasted, shelled pistachios
- ¼ cup whole wheat breadcrumbs
- One garlic clove, minced
- One shallot, minced
- ½ teaspoon dried tarragon
- One teaspoon grated lemon zest
- Sea salt, to taste (optional)
- Black pepper, to taste
- One tablespoon Dijon mustard
- One tablespoon lemon juice

Directions:

1. Warm up the oven to 400°F (205°C). Line a baking sheet with parchment paper.
2. Then place the pistachios in a food processor until they are about the size of the breadcrumbs. Mix the pistachios, breadcrumbs, garlic, shallot, tarragon, and lemon zest in a shallow dish. Sprinkle with salt (if desired) and pepper. Set aside.
3. Sprinkle the tofu with salt (if desired) and pepper. Mix the mustard and lemon juice in a small bowl and stir well.
4. Brush all over the tofu with the mustard mixture, then coat each slice with the pistachio mixture.
5. Arrange the tofu on the baking sheet. Scatter any remaining pistachio mixture over the slices.
6. Bake in the warmed oven for about 18 to 20 minutes, or until the tofu is browned and crispy.
7. Serve hot.

Nutrition: calories 159, fat 9, carbs 48, protein 10

124. Instant Savory Gigante Beans

Preparation Time: 10-30 Minutes

Cooking Time: 55 Minutes

Servings: 6

Ingredients:

- 1 lb. Gigante Beans soaked overnight
- 1/2 cup olive oil
- One onion sliced
- Two cloves garlic crushed or minced
- One red bell pepper (cut into 1/3-inch pieces)
- Two carrots, sliced
- 1/2 tsp salt and ground black pepper
- Two tomatoes peeled, grated
- 1 Tbsp celery (chopped)
- 1 tbsp tomato paste (or ketchup)
- 3/4 tsp sweet paprika
- 1 tsp oregano
- 1 cup vegetable broth

Directions:

1. Soak Gigante beans overnight.
2. Press the SAUTÉ button on your Instant Pot and heat the oil.
3. Sauté onion, garlic, sweet pepper, carrots with a pinch of salt for 3 - 4 minutes; stir occasionally.
4. Add rinsed Gigante beans into your Instant Pot along with all remaining ingredients and stir well.
5. Latch lid into place and set on the MANUAL setting for 25 minutes.
6. When the beep sounds, quick release the pressure by pressing Cancel and twisting the steam handle to the Venting position.
7. Taste and adjust seasonings to taste.
8. Serve warm or cold.
9. Keep refrigerated.

Nutrition: calories 232, fat 18, carbs 21, protein 9

125. Instant Turmeric Risotto

Preparation Time: 10-30 Minutes

Cooking Time: 40 Minutes

Servings: 4

Ingredients:

- 4 Tbsp olive oil
- 1 cup onion
- 1 tsp minced garlic
- 2 cups long-grain rice
- 3 cups vegetable broth
- 1/2 tsp paprika (smoked)
- 1/2 tsp turmeric
- 1/2 tsp nutmeg
- 2 Tbsp fresh basil leaves chopped
- Salt and ground black pepper to taste

Directions:

1. Press the SAUTÉ button on your Instant Pot and heat oil.
2. Sauté the onion and garlic with a pinch of salt until softened.
3. Add the rice and all leftover ingredients and stir well.
4. Lock the lid into place and set on and select the RICE button for 10 minutes.
5. Press Cancel when the timer beeps and carefully flip the Quick Release valve to let the pressure out.
6. Taste and adjust seasonings to taste.
7. Serve.

Nutrition: calories 154, fat 10, carbs 18, protein 9

126. Nettle Soup with Rice

Preparation Time: 10-30 Minutes

Cooking Time: 40 Minutes

Servings: 5

Ingredients:

- 3 Tbsp of olive oil
- Two onions finely chopped
- Two cloves garlic finely chopped
- Salt and freshly ground black pepper
- Four medium potatoes cut into cubes
- 1 cup of rice
- 1 Tbsp arrowroot
- 2 cups vegetable broth
- 2 cups of water
- One bunch of young nettle leaves packed
- 1/2 cup fresh parsley finely chopped
- 1 tsp cumin

Directions:

1. Heat olive oil in a large pot.
2. Sauté onion and garlic with a pinch of salt until softened.
3. Add potato, rice, and arrowroot; sauté for 2 to 3 minutes.
4. Pour broth and water, stir well, cover and cook over medium heat for about 20 minutes.
5. Cook for about 30 to 45 minutes.
6. Add young nettle leaves, parsley, and cumin; stir and cook for 5 to 7 minutes.
7. Move the soup to a blender and blend until combined well.
8. Taste and adjust salt and pepper.
9. Serve hot.

Nutrition: calories 419, fat 1, carbs 18, protein 11

127. Okra with Grated Tomatoes

Preparation Time: 10-30 Minutes

Cooking Time: 3 Hours and 10 Minutes

Servings: 4

Ingredients:

- 2 lbs. fresh okra cleaned
- Two onions finely chopped
- Two cloves garlic finely sliced
- Two carrots sliced
- Two ripe tomatoes grated
- 1 cup of water
- 4 Tbsp olive oil
- Salt and ground black pepper
- 1 tbsp fresh parsley finely chopped

Directions:

1. Add okra in your Crock-Pot: sprinkle with a pinch of salt and pepper.
2. Add in chopped onion, garlic, carrots, and grated tomatoes; stir well.
3. Pour water and oil, season with the salt, pepper, and give a good stir.
4. Cover and cook on LOW for 2-4 hours or until tender.
5. Open the lid and add fresh parsley; stir.
6. Taste and adjust salt and pepper.
7. Serve hot.

Nutrition: calories 223, fat 13, carbs 9, protein 14

128. Oven-Baked Smoked Lentil Burgers

Preparation Time: 10-30 Minutes

Cooking Time: 1 Hour and 20 Minutes

Servings: 6

Ingredients:

- 1 1/2 cups dried lentils
- 3 cups of water
- Salt and ground black pepper to taste
- 2 Tbsp olive oil
- One onion finely diced
- Two cloves minced garlic
- 1 cup button mushrooms sliced
- 2 Tbsp tomato paste
- 1/2 tsp fresh basil finely chopped
- 1 cup chopped almonds
- 3 tsp balsamic vinegar
- 3 Tbsp coconut amino
- 1 tsp liquid smoke
- 3/4 cup silken tofu soft
- 3/4 cup corn starch

Directions:

1. Cook lentils in salted water until tender or for about 30-35 minutes; rinse, drain, and set aside.
2. Heat oil in a frying skillet and sauté onion, garlic, and mushrooms for 4 to 5 minutes; stir occasionally.
3. Stir in the tomato paste, salt, basil, salt, and black pepper; cook for 2 to 3 minutes.
4. Stir in almonds, vinegar, coconut amino, liquid smoke, and lentils.
5. Remove from heat and stir in blended tofu and corn starch.
6. Keep stirring until all ingredients combined well.
7. Form mixture into patties and refrigerate for an hour.
8. Preheat oven to 350 F.
9. Line a baking dish with parchment paper and arrange patties on the pan.
10. Bake for 20 to 25 minutes.
11. Serve hot with buns, green salad, tomato sauce, etc.

Nutrition: calories 169, fat 1, carbs 11, protein 8

129. Powerful Spinach and Mustard Leaves Puree

Preparation Time: 10-30 Minutes

Cooking Time: 50 Minutes

Servings: 4

Ingredients:

- 2 Tbsp almond butter
- One onion finely diced
- 2 Tbsp minced garlic
- 1 tsp salt and black pepper (or to taste)
- 1 lb. mustard leaves cleaned rinsed
- 1 lb. frozen spinach thawed
- 1 tsp coriander
- 1 tsp ground cumin
- 1/2 cup almond milk

Directions:

1. Press the SAUTÉ button on your Instant Pot and heat the almond butter.
2. Sauté onion, garlic, and a pinch of salt for 2-3 minutes; stir occasionally.
3. Add spinach and the mustard greens and stir for a minute or two.
4. Season with the salt and pepper, coriander, and cumin; give a good stir.
5. Lock lid into place and set on the MANUAL setting for 15 minutes.
6. Use Quick Release - turn the valve from sealing to venting to release the pressure.
7. Move mixture to a blender, add almond milk, and blend until smooth.
8. Taste and adjust seasonings.
9. Serve.

Nutrition: calories 180, fat 1, carbs 18, protein 10

Chapter 10

VEGETABLE

130. Power Pesto Zoodles

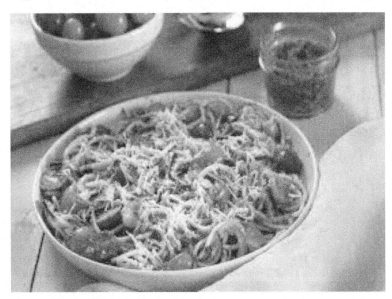

Preparation Time: 10 minutes

Cooking time: 5 minutes

Servings: 2

Ingredients:

- 2 zucchinis
- 1 avocado, peeled, pitted
- ½ cup cherry tomatoes
- 2 tablespoons walnuts

- ½ of key lime, juiced

Extra:

- ¼ teaspoon salt
- 1/8 teaspoon cayenne pepper
- 2 teaspoons grapeseed oil
- 2 tablespoons olive oil

Directions

1. Prepare the zucchini noodles and for this, cut them into thin strips by using a vegetable peeler or use a spiralizer.
2. Then take a medium skillet pan, add oil in it and when hot, add zucchini noodles in it and then cook for 3 to 5 minutes until tender-crisp.
3. Meanwhile, place the remaining ingredients in a food processor and then pulse until the creamy paste comes together.
4. When zucchini noodles have sautéed, drain and place them in a large bowl and add the blended sauce in it.
5. Add 2 tablespoons of water and then toss until well combined.
6. Garnish the zoodles with grated coconut and then serve.

Nutrition: calories 220, fat 11, carbs 18, protein 19

131. Mushroom Gravy

Preparation Time: 5 minutes

Cooking time: 12 minutes

Servings: 2

Ingredients:

- ¾ tablespoon spelt flour
- ¼ of onion, peeled, diced
- 4 ounces sliced mushrooms
- ½ cup walnut milk, homemade
- 1 tablespoon chopped walnuts

Extra:

- ¼ teaspoon salt
- 1/8 teaspoon cayenne pepper
- ½ teaspoon dried thyme
- 1 tablespoon grapeseed oil
- ¼ cup vegetable broth, homemade

Directions:

1. Take a medium skillet pan, place it over medium heat, add oil, and when hot, add onion and mushrooms, season with 1/16 teaspoon each of salt and cayenne pepper, and then cook for 4 minutes until tender.
2. Stir in spelt flour until coated, cook for 1 minute, slowly whisk in milk and vegetable broth and then season with remaining salt and cayenne pepper.
3. Switch heat to low-level, cook for 5 to 7 minutes until the sauce has thickened slightly, and then stir in walnuts and thyme.
4. Serve straight away with spelt flour bread.

Nutrition: calories 312, fat 8, carbs 18, protein 10

132. Nori Burritos

Preparation Time: 10 minutes

Cooking time: 0 minutes

Servings: 2

Ingredients:

- 1 avocado, peeled, sliced
- 1 cucumber, deseeded, cut into round slices
- 1 zucchini, sliced
- 2 teaspoons sprouted hemp seeds
- 2 nori sheets

Extra:

- 1 tablespoon tahini butter
- 2 teaspoons sesame seeds

Directions:

1. Working on one nori sheet at a time, place it on a cutting board shiny-side-down and then arrange half of each avocado, cucumber and zucchini slices and tahini on it, leaving 1-inch wide spice to the right.
2. Then start folding the sheet over the fillings from the edge that is closest to you, cut into thick slices, and then sprinkle with 1 teaspoon of sesame seeds.
3. Repeat with the remaining nori sheet, and then serve.

Nutrition: calories 210, fat 1, carbs 20, protein 11

133. Zesty Citrus Salad

Preparation Time: 5 minutes

Cooking time: 0 minutes

Servings: 2

Ingredients:

- 4 slices of onion
- ½ of avocado, peeled, pitted, sliced
- 4 ounces arugula
- 1 orange, zested, peeled, sliced
- 1 teaspoon agave syrup

Extra:

- 1/8 teaspoon salt
- 1/8 teaspoon cayenne pepper
- 2 tablespoons key lime juice
- 2 tablespoons olive oil

Directions:

1. Distribute avocado, oranges, onion, and arugula between two plates.
2. Mix together oil, salt, cayenne pepper, agave syrup, and lime juice in a small bowl and then stir until mixed.
3. Drizzle the dressing over the salad and then serve.

Nutrition: calories 276, fat 3, carbs 18, protein 11

134. Zucchini Hummus Wrap

Preparation Time: 10 minutes

Cooking time: 8 minutes

Servings: 2

Ingredients:

- ½ cup iceberg lettuce
- 1 zucchini, sliced
- 2 cherry tomatoes, sliced
- 2 spelt flour tortillas
- 4 tablespoons homemade hummus

Extra:

- ¼ teaspoon salt
- 1/8 teaspoon cayenne pepper
- 1 tablespoon grapeseed oil

Directions:

1. Take a grill pan, grease it with oil and let it preheat over medium-high heat setting.
2. Meanwhile, place zucchini slices in a large bowl, sprinkle with salt and cayenne pepper, drizzle with oil and then toss until coated.
3. Arrange zucchini slices on the grill pan and then cook for 2 to 3 minutes per side until developed grill marks.
4. Assemble tortillas and for this, heat the tortilla on the grill pan until warm and develop grill marks and spread 2 tablespoons of hummus over each tortilla.
5. Distribute grilled zucchini slices over the tortillas, top with lettuce and tomato slices, and then wrap tightly.
6. Serve straight away.

Nutrition: calories 132, fat 1, carbs 18, protein 10

135. Basil and Avocado Salad

Preparation Time: 10 minutes

Cooking time: 0 minutes

Servings: 2

Ingredients:

- ½ cup avocado, peeled, pitted, chopped
- ½ cup basil leaves
- ½ cup cherry tomatoes
- 2 cups cooked spelt noodles

Extra:

- 1 teaspoon agave syrup
- 1 tablespoon key lime juice
- 2 tablespoons olive oil

Directions:

1. Take a large bowl, place pasta in it, add tomato, avocado, and basil in it and then stir until mixed.
2. Take a small bowl, add agave syrup and salt in it, pour in lime juice and olive oil, and then whisk until combined.
3. Pour lime juice mixture over pasta, toss until combined, and then serve.

Nutrition: calories 188, fat 10, carbs 9, protein 22

136. Vegan Portobello Burgers

Preparation Time: 10 minutes

Cooking time: 20 minutes

Servings: 2

Ingredients:

- 2 Portobello mushroom caps
- ½ of avocado, sliced
- 1 cup purslane
- 2 teaspoons dried basil

- 2 tablespoons olive oil

Extra:

- ¼ teaspoon salt
- 1 teaspoon dried oregano
- ½ teaspoon cayenne pepper

Directions:

1. Switch on the oven, then set it to 425 degrees F and let it preheat.
2. Prepare the marinade and for this, take a small bowl, pour in oil, add cayenne pepper, onion powder, oregano, and basil and then stir until mixed.
3. Take a cookie sheet, line it with a foil, brush with oil, place mushroom caps on it, evenly pour the marinade over mushroom caps and then let them marinate for 10 minutes.
4. Then bake the mushroom caps for 20 minutes, flipping halfway, until tender and cooked.
5. When done, place mushroom caps on two plates, top the caps with avocado and purslane evenly and then serve.

Nutrition: calories 132, fat 13, carbs 18, protein 28

137. Grilled Romaine Lettuce Salad

Preparation Time: 10 minutes

Cooking time: 10 minutes

Servings: 2

Ingredients:

- 2 small heads of romaine lettuce, cut in half
- 1 tablespoon chopped basil
- 1 tablespoon chopped red onion
- ¼ teaspoon onion powder
- ½ tablespoon agave syrup

Extra:

- ½ teaspoon salt
- ¼ teaspoon cayenne pepper

- 2 tablespoons olive oil
- 1 tablespoon key lime juice

Directions:

1. Take a large skillet pan, place it over medium heat and when warmed, arrange lettuce heads in it, cut-side down, and then cook for 4 to 5 minutes per side until golden brown on both sides.
2. When done, transfer lettuce heads to a plate and then let them cool for 5 minutes.
3. Meanwhile, prepare the dressing and for this, place remaining ingredients in a small bowl and then stir until combined.
4. Drizzle the dressing over lettuce heads and then serve.

Nutrition: calories 190, fat 18, carbs 18, protein 32

138. Vegetable Fajitas

Preparation Time: 10 minutes

Cooking time: 8 minutes

Servings: 2

Ingredients:

- 2 Portobello mushroom caps, 1/3-inch sliced
- ¾ of red bell pepper, sliced
- ½ of onion, peeled, sliced
- ½ of key lime, juiced
- 2 spelt flour tortillas

Extra:

- 1/3 teaspoon salt
- ¼ teaspoon cayenne pepper
- ¼ teaspoon onion powder
- 1 tablespoon grapeseed oil

Directions

1. Take a medium skillet pan, place it over medium heat, add oil, and when hot, add onion and red pepper, and then cook for 2 minutes until tender-crisp.

2. Add mushrooms slices, sprinkle with all the seasoning, stir until mixed, and then cook for 5 minutes until vegetables turn soft.
3. Heat the tortilla until warm, distribute vegetables in their center, drizzle with lime juice, and then roll tightly.
4. Serve straight away.

Nutrition: calories 220, fat 23, carbs 12, protein 28

139. Appetizing Baked Apple

Preparation Time: 10 minutes

Cooking time: 55 minutes

Servings: 2

Ingredients:

- 4 apples, large, cored, sliced
- 1/8 teaspoon ground cloves
- 3 tablespoons agave syrup
- 1 tablespoon chopped walnuts

Directions

1. Switch on the oven, then set it to 350 degrees F and let it preheat.
2. Meanwhile, take a large bowl, place apple slices in it, drizzle with agave syrup and then toss until evenly coated.
3. Take a small bowl, place nuts in it, add cloves, and then stir until mixed.
4. Sprinkle nuts mixture over the apple and let it rest for 5 minutes or more until apples start releasing their juices.
5. Take a medium casserole dish, arrange apple slices on it, and then bake for 15 minutes.
6. Cover the casserole dish with foil and then continue baking for 40 minutes until bubbly.
7. Let apples cool for 10 minutes and then serve.

Nutrition: calories 184, fat 20, carbs 18, protein 26

140. Classic Banana Fries

Preparation Time: 5 minutes

Cooking time: 10 minutes

Servings: 2

Ingredients:

- 4 baby burro bananas, peeled, cut into squares
- ¼ teaspoon salt
- ½ of a medium onion, peeled, chopped
- ½ of medium green bell pepper, cored, chopped
- 2 teaspoons grapeseed oil

Extra:

- ¼ teaspoon cayenne pepper

Directions

1. Take a medium skillet pan, place it over medium-low heat, add oil, and when hot, add burro banana pieces, and then cook for 3 minutes or until beginning to brown.
2. Then turn the burro banana pieces, add remaining ingredients, stir until mixed, and then continue cooking for 5 to 7 minutes until onions have caramelized.
3. Serve straight away.

Nutrition: calories 188, fat 18, carbs 10, protein 32

141. Zoodles with Basil & Avocado Sauce

Preparation Time: 10 minutes

Cooking time: 0 minutes

Servings: 2

Ingredients:

- 2 zucchinis, spiralized into noodles
- 2 avocados, peeled, pitted
- ½ cup walnuts

- 2 cups basil leaves
- 24 cherry tomatoes, sliced

Extra:

- 1/3 teaspoon salt
- 4 tablespoons key lime juice
- ½ cup spring water

Directions:

1. Prepare the sauce and for this, place all the ingredients except for zucchini noodles and tomatoes in a food processor and then pulse until smooth.
2. Take a large bowl, place zucchini noodles in it, add tomato slices, pour in the prepared sauce, and then toss until coated.
3. Serve straight away.

Nutrition: calories 188, fat 21, carbs 10, protein 22

142. Butternut Squash and Apple Burger

Preparation Time: 10 minutes

Cooking time: 1 hour

Servings: 2

Ingredients:

- ¾ cup diced butternut squash
- ½ cup diced apples
- 1 cup cooked wild rice
- ¼ cup chopped shallots
- ½ tablespoon thyme

Extra:

- ¼ teaspoon sea salt, divided
- 1 tablespoon pumpkin seeds, unsalted
- 1 tablespoon grapeseed oil
- 2 spelt burgers, halved, toasted

Directions

1. Switch on the oven, then set it to 400 degrees F and let it preheat.
2. Meanwhile, take a cookie sheet, line it with parchment sheet, spread squash pieces on it and then sprinkle with 1/8 teaspoon salt.
3. Bake the squash for 15 minutes, then add shallots and apple, sprinkle with remaining salt, and then bake for 20 to 30 minutes until cooked.
4. When done, let the vegetable mixture cool for 15 minutes, transfer it into a food processor, add thyme and then pulse until a chunky mixture comes together.
5. Add pumpkin seeds and cooked wild rice, pulse until combined, and then tip the mixture in a bowl.
6. Taste the mixture to adjust and then shape it into two patties.
7. Take a skillet pan, place it over medium heat, add oil and when hot, place patties in it and then cook for 5 to 7 minutes per side until browned.
8. Sandwich patties in burger buns and then serve.

Nutrition: calories 210, fat 13, carbs 18, protein 21

143. Kale and Avocado Dish

Preparation Time: 5 minutes

Cooking time: 0 minutes

Servings: 2

Ingredients

- 1 bundle of kale, cut into thin strips
- 1 small white onion, peeled, chopped
- 12 cherry tomatoes, chopped
- 1 tablespoon salt
- 1 avocado, peeled, pitted, sliced

Directions

1. Take a large bowl, place kale strips in it, sprinkle with salt, and then massage for 2 minutes.
2. Cover the bowl with a plastic wrap or its lid, let it rest for a minimum of 30 minutes, and then stir in onion and tomatoes until well combined.

3. Let the salad sit for 5 minutes, add avocado slices, and then serve.

Nutrition: calories 110, fat 19, carbs 7, protein 21

Chapter 11

DINNER RECIPES

144. Roasted Sweet Potatoes

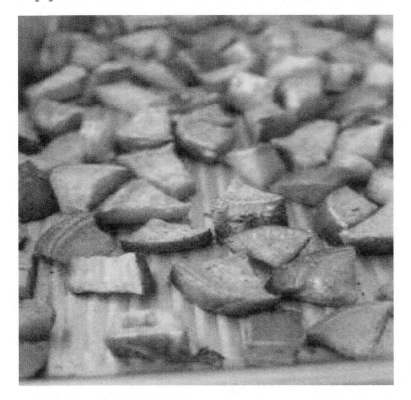

Preparation time: 10 minutes

Cooking time: 45 minutes

Servings: 4

Ingredients:

- 2 sweet potatoes, peeled and cubed
- 2½ tablespoons avocado oil
- A pinch of salt and black pepper
- 1 garlic clove, minced
- Juice of 1 lime
- 4 tablespoons water

Directions:

1. Spread the potatoes on a lined baking sheet and combine with the rest of the ingredients.
2. Cook at 400 degrees F for 45 minutes and serve for lunch.

Nutrition: calories 222, fat 6, carbs 15, protein 7

145. Lemony Carrot Soup

Preparation time: 10 minutes

Cooking time: 40 minutes

Servings: 4

Ingredients:

- 2 cups carrots, sliced
- 1 tablespoon olive oil
- 1 yellow onion, chopped
- 1½ cups kale, chopped
- 1 cup plum tomatoes, cubed
- 3 garlic cloves, minced
- A pinch of salt and black pepper
- 4 teaspoons fresh grated ginger
- 4 cups water
- 1 teaspoon sweet paprika
- 2 teaspoons ground turmeric
- Juice of 1 lemon
- Zest of ½ lemon, grated

Directions:

1. Heat up a pot with the oil over medium heat, add the onion and garlic, and cook for 5 minutes.
2. Add the carrots and the other ingredients, stir and simmer for 35 minutes more.
3. Divide into bowls and serve.

Nutrition: calories 271, fat 8, carbs 8,3, protein 8

146. Burrito Bowls

Preparation time: 10 minutes

Cooking time: 0 minutes

Servings: 1

Ingredients:

- ¼ cup spinach leaves, torn
- 1 tablespoon chives, chopped
- 1 tablespoon chopped red bell pepper
- 1 teaspoon olive oil
- 3 cherry tomatoes, halved
- 1 tablespoon chopped parsley
- 1 red cabbage, shredded
- Juice of 1 lime

Directions:

1. In a bowl, mix the spinach with the chives and the other ingredients, toss, and serve for lunch.

Nutrition*:* calories 207, fat 3.8, carbs 6, protein 4.4

147. Mixed Beans Bowls

Preparation time: 10 minutes

Cooking time: 40 minutes

Servings: 4

Ingredients:

- 1 cup pinto beans, rinsed
- 1 cup red beans, rinsed
- 1 cup white beans, rinsed
- 1 cup soybeans, rinsed
- 1 yellow onions, chopped
- 1 tablespoon avocado oil
- 1 cup cherry tomatoes, halved
- 1 cup baby spinach
- 1 small jalapeno pepper, minced
- 2 teaspoons lime juice
- Zest of 1 lime, grated
- Salt and black pepper to the taste
- 1 teaspoon turmeric powder

Directions:

1. Heat up a pan with the oil over medium heat, add the onion, jalapeno and turmeric and cook for 5 minutes.
2. Add the rest of the ingredients, stir and simmer over medium heat for 35 minutes stirring from time to time.
3. Divide into bowls and serve for lunch.

Nutrition: calories 320, fat 12, carbs 12, protein 7

148. Bell Peppers Soup

Preparation time: 10 minutes

Cooking time: 40 minutes

Servings: 4

Ingredients:

- 4 shallots, chopped
- 3 carrots, chopped
- 1-pound mixed bell peppers, cut into strips
- A pinch of salt and black pepper
- 1 teaspoon hot paprika
- 4 cups water
- 1½ cups cauliflower florets, chopped
- 2 cups kale, chopped
- 2 tablespoons avocado oil
- 1 cup cherry tomatoes, chopped
- 1 teaspoon oregano, dried

Directions:

1. Heat up a pot with the oil over medium-high heat, add the shallots and carrots and cook for 5 minutes.
2. Add the peppers and the other ingredients, stir, simmer over medium heat for 35 minutes more, ladle into bowls and serve for lunch.

Nutrition: calories 210, fat 4.4, carbs 14, protein 6.3

149. Carrots and Onion Mix

Preparation time: 10 minutes

Cooking time: 25 minutes

Servings: 4

Ingredients:

- 1-pound baby carrots, trimmed
- 3 garlic cloves, minced

- 1 cup pearl onions, peeled
- Salt and black pepper to the taste
- 2 tablespoons coconut oil, melted
- 2 tablespoons chopped tarragon
- ¼ cup chopped parsley
- Juice of 1 lemon
- 1 tablespoon chopped thyme
- 1 cup cherry tomatoes, halved

Directions:

1. Heat up a pan with the oil over medium-high heat, add the onions and garlic and cook for 5 minutes.
2. Add the rest of the ingredients, stir, cook for 20 minutes more, divide between plates, and serve.

Nutrition: calories 173, fat 3, carbs 9, protein 5

150. Mixed Berry Crisp

Preparation Time: 10 Minutes

Cooking Time: 0

Servings: 4

Ingredients:

- 1 ½ cups mixed berries (I used raspberries, blueberries, and blackberries)
- ½ tablespoon cornstarch
- 2 tablespoons butter, room temperature
- ¼ cup old fashioned oats, plus 1 tablespoon old fashioned oats
- ¼ cup brown sugar
- 3 tablespoons flour
- ¼ teaspoon cinnamon
- ¼ teaspoon nutmeg
- 1 tablespoon water

Directions:

1. Preheat oven to 375 degrees.
2. In a small bowl, combine the butter, oats, brown sugar, flour, cinnamon, and nutmeg. Mix lightly with a fork until the mixture is crumbly.
3. Top the berries with the crisp mixture. Sprinkle the top of the crisp with water.
4. Bake for 25 minutes or until the fruit is bubbling and the topping is slightly browned.
5. Serve with ice cream, frozen yogurt, or whipped cream.

Nutrition: calories 226, fat 21, carbs 18, protein 11

151. Strawberry Daiquiri

Preparation Time: 10 Minutes

Cooking Time: 24 Minutes

Servings: 4

Ingredients:

- 1 (10-ounce) can frozen strawberry daiquiri concentrate
- 1 ½ cups frozen strawberries
- 1 cup ice cube

Directions:

1. Combine all ingredients together in a blender until all the ice is crushed.
2. Add more or fewer ice cubes for the right texture.

Nutrition: calories 116, fat 21, carbs 8, protein 4

152. Virgin White Sangria

Preparation Time: 5 Minutes

Cooking Time: 4 Minutes

Servings: 1

Ingredients:

- 4 cups ocean spray white cranberry juice with Splenda

- 2 cups fresh fruit, sliced
- 1 cup diet lemon-lime soda
- 1 lime, juice of

Directions:

1. Combine all the ingredients except the soda in a large pitcher and chill for at least 1 hour.
2. When serving, add the soda. Serve with a pretty fruit garnish.

Nutrition: calories 129, fat 23, carbs 8, protein 18

153. Wow Cola Chicken

Preparation Time: 15 Minutes

Cooking Time: 14 Minutes

Servings: 1

Ingredients:

- 16 ounces boneless chicken breasts
- 1 (12 ounce) can diet cola
- 1 cup ketchup

Directions:

1. Place chicken in crockpot and then top with ketchup and then pour cola over all.
2. Cook on low for 6-8 hours.

Nutrition: calories 218, fat 19, carbs 18, protein 28

154. Warm Apple Delight

Preparation Time: 5 Minutes

Cooking Time: 4 Minutes

Servings: 1

Ingredients:

- 2 red apples, cored & cut in half
- 1 (375 ml) can flavored diet cola (cherry or strawberry suggested)

- 1 pinch Splenda sugar substitute or 1 pinch Equal sugar substitute
- 1 pinch cinnamon

Directions:

1. Place the apple in a baking dish, skin side down and pour the cola over.
2. Sprinkle with sweetener & cinnamon.
3. Bake in a pre-heated oven at 180.C for 25-30 minutes.

Nutrition: calories 156, fat 22, carbs 5, protein 4

155. Orange Dream Cake

Preparation Time: 5 Minutes

Cooking Time: 4 Minutes

Servings: 1

Ingredients:

- 2 egg whites
- 6 ounces sugar-free orange gelatin, divided (2 pkgs)
- 1 cup hot water
- 1 cup cold water

TOPPING

- 3 ½ ounces fat-free sugar-free vanilla pudding mix
- 1 cup nonfat milk
- 1 teaspoon vanilla extract
- 8 ounces Cool Whip Free, thawed

Directions

1. Mix Cake mix, soda, and egg whites together.
2. Pour batter into a 9 X 13-inch pan.
3. Bake as directed on box.
4. Pour gelatin mixture over top of the cake.
5. Refrigerate for 2 to 3 hours.

Nutrition: calories 109, fat 28, carbs 18, protein 19

156. Delicious Low-Cal Smoothie

Preparation Time: 5 Minutes

Cooking Time: 4 Minutes

Servings: 1

Ingredients:

- 1 cup frozen raspberries
- 1 ½ cups frozen strawberries
- 1 cup pineapple
- 355 ml diet Sprite

Directions:

1. Blend on high power until smooth.
2. Serve in your favorite glasses, either with spoons or straws.

Nutrition: calories 126, fat 19, carbs 7, protein 11

Chapter 12

SNACKS & BREAD

157. Spinach and Sesame Crackers

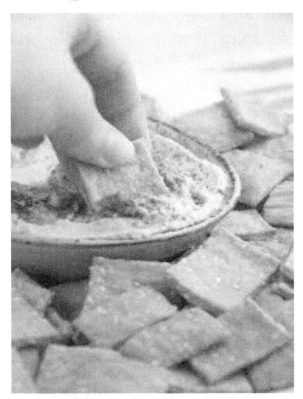

Preparation Time: 5 minutes

Cooking Time: 15 minutes

Servings: 4

Ingredients:

- 2 tablespoons white sesame seeds
- 1 cup fresh spinach, washed
- 1 2/3 cups of all-purpose flour
- 1/2 cup of water
- 1/2 teaspoon baking powder
- 1 teaspoon olive oil
- 1 teaspoon of salt

Directions:

1. Transfer the spinach to a blender with a half cup of water and blend until smooth.
2. Add 2 tablespoons white sesame seeds, ½ teaspoon baking powder, 1 2/3 cups all-purpose flour, and 1 teaspoon salt to a bowl and stir well until combined. Add in 1 teaspoon olive oil and spinach water. Mix again and knead by using your hands until you obtain a smooth dough.
3. If the made dough is too gluey, then add more flour.
4. Using your parchment paper lightly roll out the dough as thin as possible. Cut into squares with a pizza cutter.
5. Bake in a preheated oven at 400° for about 15to 20 minutes. Once done, let cool and then serve.

Nutrition: calories 190, fat 17, carbs 8, protein 11

158. Mini Nacho Pizzas

Preparation Time: 5 minutes

Cooking Time: 10 minutes

Servings: 4

Ingredients:

- 1/4 cup refried beans, vegan
- 2 tablespoons tomato, diced
- 2 English muffins, split in half
- 1/4 cup onion, sliced
- 1/3 cup vegan cheese, shredded

- 1 small jalapeno, sliced
- 1/3 cup roasted tomato salsa
- 1/2 avocado, diced and tossed in lemon juice

Directions:

1. Add the refried beans/salsa onto the muffin bread. Sprinkle with shredded vegan cheese followed by the veggie toppings.
2. Transfer to a baking sheet and place in a preheated oven at 350 to 400 F on a top rack.
3. Put into the oven for 10 minutes and then broil for 2minutes, so that the top becomes bubbly.
4. Take out from the oven and let them cool at room temperature.
5. Top with avocado. Enjoy!

Nutrition: calories 112, fat 23, carbs 18, protein 28

159. Pizza Sticks

Preparation Time: 10 minutes

Cooking Time: 30 minutes

Servings: 16 sticks

Ingredients:

- 5 tablespoons tomato sauce
- Few pinches of dried basil
- 1 block extra firm tofu
- 2 tablespoon + 2 teaspoon nutritional yeast

Directions:

1. Cape the tofu in a paper tissue and put a cutting board on top, place something heavy on top and drain for about 10 to 15 minutes.
2. In the meantime, line your baking sheet with parchment paper. Cut the tofu into 16 equal pieces and place them on a baking sheet.
3. Spread each pizza stick with a teaspoon of marinara sauce.
4. Sprinkle each stick with a half teaspoon of yeast, followed by basil on top.
5. Bake in a preheated oven at 425 F for about 28 to 30 minutes. Serve and enjoy!

Nutrition: calories 190, fat 23, carbs 8, protein 19

160. Raw Broccoli Poppers

Preparation Time: 2 minutes

Cooking Time: 8 minutes

Servings: 4

Ingredients:

- 1/8 cup of water
- 1/8 teaspoon of fine sea salt
- 4 cups broccoli florets, washed and cut into 1-inch pieces
- 1/4 teaspoon turmeric powder
- 1 cup unsalted cashews, soaked overnight or at least 3-4 hours and drained
- 1/4 teaspoon onion powder
- 1 red bell pepper, seeded and
- 2 heaping tablespoons nutritional
- 2 tablespoons lemon juice

Directions:

1. Transfer the drained cashews to a high-speed blender and pulse for about 30 seconds. Add in the chopped pepper and pulse again for 30 seconds.
2. Add some 2 tablespoons of lemon juice, 1/8 cup of water, 2 heaping tablespoons of nutritional yeast, ¼ teaspoon of onion powder, 1/8 teaspoon of fine sea salt, and 1/4 teaspoon of turmeric powder. Pulse for about 45 seconds until smooth.
3. Handover the broccoli into a bowl and add in chopped cheesy cashew mixture. Toss well until coated.
4. Transfer the pieces of broccoli to the trays of a yeast dehydrator.
5. Follow the dehydrator's instructions and dehydrate for about 8 minutes at 125 F or until crunchy.

Nutrition: calories 134, fat 18, carbs 6, protein 9

161. Blueberry Cauliflower

Preparation Time: 2 minutes

Cooking Time: 5 minutes

Servings: 1

Ingredients:

- ¼ cup of frozen strawberries
- 2 teaspoons maple syrup
- ¾ cup unsweetened cashew milk
- 1 teaspoon vanilla extract
- ½ cup of plain cashew yogurt
- 5 tablespoons powdered peanut butter
- ¾ cup of frozen wild blueberries
- ½ cup of cauliflower florets, coarsely chopped

Directions:

1. Add all the smoothie ingredients to a high-speed blender.
2. Blitz to combine until smooth.
3. Pour into a chilled glass and serve.

Nutrition: calories 219, fat 11, carbs 8, protein 17

162. Candied Ginger

Preparation Time: 10 minutes

Cooking Time: 40 minutes

Servings: 3 to 5

Ingredients:

- 2 1/2 cups salted pistachios, shelled
- 1 1/4 teaspoons powdered ginger
- 3 tablespoons pure maple syrup

Directions:

1. Add 1 1/4 teaspoons powdered ginger to a bowl with pistachios. Stir well until combined. There should be no lumps.

2. Drizzle with 3 tablespoons of maple syrup and stir well.
3. Transfer to a baking sheet lined with parchment paper and spread evenly.
4. Cook into a preheated oven at 275 F for about 20 minutes.
5. Take out from the oven, stir, and cook for a further 10 to 15 minutes.
6. Let it cool for about a few minutes until crispy. Enjoy!

163. Chia Crackers

Preparation Time: 20 minutes

Cooking Time: 1 hour

Servings: 24-26 crackers

Ingredients:

- 1/2 cup of pecans, chopped
- 1/2 cup of chia seeds
- 1/2 teaspoon cayenne pepper
- 1 cup of water
- 1/4 cup of nutritional yeast
- 1/2 cup of pumpkin seeds
- 1/4 cup of ground flax
- Salt and pepper, to taste

Directions:

1. Mix around 1/2 cup chia seeds and 1 cup water. Keep it aside.
2. Take another bowl and combine all the remaining ingredients. Combine well and stir in the chia water mixture until you obtain dough.
3. Transfer the dough onto a baking sheet and rollout (¼" thick).
4. Transfer into a preheated oven at 325°F and bake for about half an hour.
5. Take out from the oven, flip over the dough, and cut it into the desired cracker shape/squares.
6. Spread and back again for a further half an hour, or until crispy and browned.
7. Once done, take out from the oven and let them cool at room temperature. Enjoy!

Nutrition: calories 90, fat 3, carbs 18, protein 10

164. Orange- Spiced Pumpkin Hummus

Preparation Time: 2 minutes

Cooking Time: 5 minutes

Servings: 4 cups

Ingredients:

- 1 tablespoon maple syrup
- 1/2 teaspoon salt
- 1 can (16oz.) garbanzo beans,
- 1/8 teaspoon ginger or nutmeg
- 1 cup of canned pumpkin
- 1/8 teaspoon cinnamon
- 1/4 cup of tahini
- 1 tablespoon fresh orange juice
- A pinch of orange zest, for garnish
- 1 tablespoon apple cider vinegar

Directions:

1. Mix all the ingredients to a food processor blender and blend until slightly chunky.
2. Serve right away and enjoy it!

165. Cinnamon Maple Sweet Potato Bites

Preparation Time: 5 minutes

Cooking Time: 25 minutes

Servings: 3 to 4

Ingredients:

- ½ teaspoon corn-starch
- 1 teaspoon cinnamon
- 4 medium sweet potatoes, then peeled, and cut into bite-size cubes
- 2 to 3 tablespoons maple syrup
- 3 tablespoons butter, melted

Directions:

1. Transfer the potato cubes to a Ziploc bag and add in 3 tablespoons of melted butter. Seal and shake well until the potato cubes are coated with butter.
2. Add in the remaining ingredients and shake again.
3. Transfer the potato cubes to a parchment-lined baking sheet. Cubes shouldn't be stacked on one another.
4. Sprinkle with cinnamon, if needed, and bake in a preheated oven at 425°F for about 25 to 30 minutes, stirring once during cooking.
5. Once done, take them out and stand at room temperature. Enjoy!

Nutrition: calories 188, fat 6, carbs 9, protein 18

166. Cheesy Kale Chips

Preparation Time: 3 minutes

Cooking Time: 12 minutes

Servings: 4

Ingredients:

- 3 tablespoons nutritional yeast
- 1 head curly kale, washed, ribs
- 3/4 teaspoon garlic powder
- 1 tablespoon olive oil
- 1 teaspoon onion powder
- Salt, to taste

Directions:

1. Line cookie sheets with parchment paper.
2. Drain the kale leaves and spread on a paper removed and leaves torn into a chip-towel. Then, kindly transfer the leaves to a bowl and sized pieces. Add in 1 teaspoon of onion powder, 3 tablespoons of nutritional yeast, 1 tablespoon of olive oil, and ¾ teaspoon of garlic powder. Mix with your hands.
3. Spread the kale onto prepared cookie sheets. They shouldn't touch each other.
4. Bake in a preheated oven for about 350 F for about 10 to 12 minutes.

5. Once crisp, take out from the oven, and sprinkle with a bit of salt. Serve and enjoy!

Nutrition: calories 286, fat 4, carbs 18, protein 10

167. Broccoli Bowls

Preparation time: 10 minutes

Cooking time: 15 minutes

Servings: 2

Ingredients:

- 1-pound broccoli florets
- 1 cup avocado, peeled, pitted, and cubed
- 1 red onion, chopped
- 1 red bell pepper, chopped
- 1 tablespoon coconut oil, melted
- 1 tablespoon avocado oil
- 1 teaspoon lemon juice
- Salt and black pepper to the taste
- ½ teaspoon ground turmeric

Directions:

1. Heat up a pan with the oil over medium heat, add the broccoli, avocado, and the other ingredients, stir and cook for 15 minutes.
2. Divide into bowls and serve as an appetizer.

Nutrition: calories 238, fat 8, carbs 10.3, protein 6.9

168. Celery Appetizer

Preparation time: 10 minutes

Cooking time: 30 minutes

Servings: 2

Ingredients:

- Juice of 1 lemon
- 6 celery stalks, chopped
- 2 teaspoons olive oil
- Salt and black pepper to the taste
- 4 tablespoons chopped parsley

Directions:

1. Spread the celery on a lined baking sheet, add the rest of the ingredients, toss, and cook at 390 degrees F for 30 minutes.
2. Serve as an appetizer.

Nutrition: calories 210, fat 6, carbs 6, protein 13

169. Seeds Mix

Preparation time: 10 minutes

Cooking time: 30 minutes

Servings: 4

Ingredients:

- 1 cup sunflower seeds
- 1 cup pumpkin seeds
- A pinch of salt and black pepper
- 1 teaspoon ground thyme
- A drizzle of olive oil

Directions:

1. Spread the seeds on a lined baking sheet, add the rest of the ingredients, toss, and bake at 350 degrees F for 30 minutes.
2. Serve as a snack.

Nutrition: calories 90, fat 2, carbs 1, protein 1

170. Herbed Endive Mix

Preparation time: 10 minutes

Cooking time: 10 minutes

Servings: 4

Ingredients:

- 2 tablespoons olive oil
- Salt and black pepper to the taste
- 2 tablespoons lime juice
- 3 endives, shredded
- 3 tablespoons chopped parsley
- 2 teaspoons chopped mint
- 1 tablespoon chopped tarragon

Directions:

1. On a lined baking sheet, mix the endives with the rest of the ingredients and toss.
2. Bake in the oven at 400 degrees F for 10 minutes.
3. Serve as an appetizer.

Nutrition: calories 160, fat 7, carbs 3, protein 3

171. Beet Chips

Preparation time: 10 minutes

Cooking time: 45 minutes

Servings: 4

Ingredients:

- 2 big beets, peeled and thinly sliced
- Juice of 1 lemon
- 1 Serrano chili pepper, chopped
- ½ teaspoon fresh grated ginger
- ¼ teaspoon minced garlic
- A pinch of salt and black pepper

- 2 tablespoons avocado oil
- ¼ cup chopped cilantro

Directions:

1. Spread the chips on a lined baking sheet, add the rest of the ingredients, toss, and bake at 390 degrees F for 45 minutes.
2. Serve as a snack.

Nutrition: calories 160, fat 3, carbs 5, protein 5

172. Avocado and Radish Salsa

Preparation time: 10 minutes

Cooking time: 0 minutes

Servings: 4

Ingredients:

- 2 small avocados, pitted, peeled, and chopped
- 2 cups radishes, cubed
- 1 cup cucumber, cubed
- Juice of 1 lemon
- 1 tablespoon avocado oil
- 1 tablespoon chives, chopped
- 1 tablespoon cilantro, chopped

Directions:

1. In a bowl, mix the avocados with the radishes and the other ingredients, toss, and serve.

Nutrition: calories 220, fat 6, carbs 12, protein 6

173. Tomato Platter

Preparation time: 10 minutes

Cooking time: 20 minutes

Servings: 6

Ingredients:

- 2 pounds cherry tomatoes, halved
- 1 teaspoon crushed red pepper flakes
- 3 garlic cloves, minced
- 1 handful chopped parsley
- 1 teaspoon curry powder
- 1 teaspoon sweet paprika
- Salt and black pepper to the taste
- 1 tablespoon avocado oil

Directions:

1. Spread the tomatoes on a lined baking sheet, add the rest of the ingredients, toss and roast at 400 degrees F for 20 minutes.
2. Serve as an appetizer.

Nutrition: calories 170, fat 3.4, carbs 6, protein 5.5

174. Cauliflower and Broccoli Bites

Preparation time: 10 minutes

Cooking time: 20 minutes

Servings: 4

Ingredients:

- 1 cup cauliflower florets
- 1 cup broccoli florets
- 2 tablespoons avocado oil
- 2 tablespoons green onions, chopped
- 1 teaspoon sweet paprika
- 1 tablespoon lemon juice
- A pinch of salt

Directions:

1. Spread the broccoli and cauliflower on a lined baking sheet, add the rest of the ingredients, toss, and bake at 400 degrees F for 20 minutes.
2. Divide into bowls and serve as a snack.

Nutrition: calories 180, fat 6.6, carbs 6, protein 5.2

175. Avocado Bites

Preparation time: 10 minutes

Cooking time: 0 minutes

Servings: 2

Ingredients:

- 2 avocados, peeled, pitted, and cubed
- 2 tablespoons sweet paprika
- juice of 1 lemon
- 1 teaspoon basil, dried
- 1 teaspoon oregano, dried
- Salt and black pepper to the taste
- 1 tablespoon olive oil

Directions:

1. In a bowl, mix the avocado bites with the paprika and the other ingredients, toss, divide into bowls and serve as a snack.

Nutrition: calories 60, fat 3, carbs 4.2, protein 4.4

176. Chives Dip

Preparation time: 10 minutes

Cooking time: 0 minutes

Servings: 4

Ingredients:

- 2 cups chives, chopped
- 1/2 cup almond milk
- ¼ cup chopped carrot
- ¼ cup chopped red onion
- Salt and black pepper to the taste
- 1 teaspoon sweet paprika

Directions:

1. In a blender, mix the chives with the carrot and the other ingredients and blend well.
2. Divide into bowls and serve.

Nutrition: calories 210, fat 3.4, carbs 6.4, protein 6

177. Stuffed Avocado

Preparation time: 10 minutes

Cooking time: 0 minutes

Servings: 2

Ingredients:

- 2 avocados, halved, pitted and flesh scooped out
- ¼ cup chives, chopped
- ½ cup carrot, grated
- ½ cup kale, chopped
- 1 teaspoon dried thyme
- A pinch of salt and black pepper
- ¼ teaspoon cayenne pepper
- 1 teaspoon paprika
- Salt and black pepper to the taste
- 2 tablespoons lemon juice

Directions:

1. In a bowl, mix the chives with carrots, avocado flesh, and the other ingredients except for the avocado shells and stir well.
2. Stuff the avocado skins with this mix, arrange them on a platter, and serve as an appetizer.

Nutrition: calories 160, fat 10, carbs 4,2, protein 5.5

178. Radish Chips

Preparation time: 10 minutes

Cooking time: 20 minutes

Servings: 4

Ingredients:

- 2 teaspoons avocado oil
- 15 radishes, sliced
- A pinch of salt and black pepper
- 1 tablespoon chopped chives

Directions:

1. Arrange radish slices on a lined baking sheet, add the other ingredients, toss, and place in the oven at 375 degrees F.
2. Bake for 10 minutes on each side, divide into bowls, and serve cold.

Nutrition: calories 30, fat 1, fiber 2, carbs 7, protein 1

179. Avocado Cream

Preparation time: 10 minutes

Cooking time: 10 minutes

Servings: 4

Ingredients:

- 2 avocados, pitted, peeled, and chopped
- 1 cup almond milk
- 2 scallions, chopped
- Salt and black pepper to the taste
- 2 tablespoons coconut oil
- 1 tablespoon chives, chopped

Directions:

1. Heat up a pot with the coconut oil over medium heat.
2. Add scallions and avocado and cook for 2 minutes.

3. Add the rest of the ingredients, cook for 8 minutes more, blend with an immersion blender, divide into bowls, and serve.

Nutrition: calories 162, fat 4.4, carbs 6, protein 6

180. Chives Chutney

Preparation time: 10 minutes

Cooking time: 20 minutes

Servings: 10

Ingredients:

- 1 teaspoon cumin seeds
- 1 tablespoon avocado oil
- 1 cup chives, chopped
- ½ cup water
- 1 cup cherry tomatoes, cubed
- ½ teaspoon garam masala
- 1 teaspoon ground ginger
- ½ teaspoon cayenne pepper

Directions:

1. Heat up a pan with the oil over medium heat, add the chives and cumin and cook for 5 minutes.
2. Add the rest of the ingredients, simmer the mixture over medium heat for 15 minutes more, divide into bowls, and serve cold.

Nutrition: calories 120, fat 4,4, carbs 5, protein 6

181. Onion Bowls

Preparation time: 10 minutes

Cooking time: 15 minutes

Servings: 4

Ingredients:

- 1 tablespoon avocado oil
- 3 red onions, cut into thin strips
- A pinch of salt and black pepper
- 1 teaspoon sweet paprika
- 1 teaspoon dried basil
- 1 teaspoon oregano, dried

Directions:

1. Heat up a pan with the oil over medium heat, add the onions and cook for 5 minutes.
2. Add the rest of the ingredients, stir, cook for 10 minutes more, divide into bowls, and serve as a snack

Nutrition: calories 127, fat 4, carbs 6, protein 4.4

182. Chia Crackers

Preparation time: 10 minutes

Cooking time: 35 minutes

Servings: 12

Ingredients:

- 1 cup ice water
- 1 cup ground chia seeds
- 2 tablespoons avocado oil
- 2 tablespoons flaxseeds
- ¼ teaspoon dried oregano
- ¼ teaspoon turmeric powder
- ¼ teaspoon sweet paprika
- Salt and black pepper to the taste
- ¼ teaspoon basil, dried

Directions:

1. In a bowl, mix chia seeds with the rest of the ingredients.
2. Stir until you obtain a firm mix then spread it on a baking sheet and place in the oven at 350 degrees F and bake for 35 minutes.
3. Remove from the oven and set aside to cool down.
4. Cut into medium crackers and serve as a snack.

Nutrition: calories 50, fat 3, carbs 5, protein 2

183. Cilantro Guacamole

Preparation time: 3 hours

Cooking time: 0 minutes

Servings: 4

Ingredients:

- 2 avocados, pitted, peeled, and chopped
- ½ cup chopped cilantro
- Juice and zest of 1 lemon
- 1 cup almond milk

Directions:

1. In a blender, mix the avocados with cilantro and the other ingredients, blend and serve.

Nutrition: calories 150, fat 7, carbs 8, protein 4

Chapter 13

LUNCH AND ENTRÉES

184. Green Bean Casserole

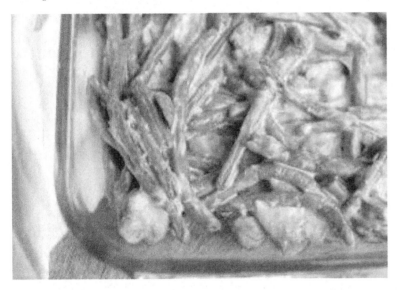

Preparation time: 20 minutes

Cooking Time: 20 minutes.

Servings: 6

Ingredients:

For Onion Slices:

- ½ cup yellow onion, sliced very thinly
- ¼ cup almond flour
- 1/8 tsp garlic powder

- Sea salt and freshly ground black pepper, to taste

For Casserole:

- 1 lb. fresh green beans, trimmed
- 1 tbsp olive oil
- 8 oz fresh cremini mushrooms, sliced
- ½ cup yellow onion, sliced thinly
- 1/8 tsp garlic powder
- Sea salt and freshly ground black pepper, to taste
- 1 tsp fresh thyme, chopped
- ½ cup homemade vegetable broth
- ½ cup coconut cream

Directions:

2. Preheat the oven to 350 degrees F.
3. For onion slices, place all the ingredients in a bowl and toss them to coat the onion well.
4. Arrange the onion slices onto a large baking sheet in a single layer and set it aside.
5. In a pan of salted boiling water, add the green beans and cook for about 5 minutes.
6. Drain the green beans and transfer them into a bowl of ice water.
7. Again, drain well and transfer them again into a large bowl. Set them aside.
8. In a large skillet, heat oil over medium-high heat and sauté the mushrooms, onion, garlic powder, salt, and black pepper for about 2-3 minutes.
9. Stir in the thyme and broth and cook for about 3-5 minutes or until all the liquid is absorbed.
10. Remove from the heat and transfer the mushroom mixture into the bowl with the green beans.
11. Add the coconut cream and stir to combine well.
12. Transfer the mixture into a 10-inch casserole dish.
13. Place the casserole dish and baking sheet of onion slices into the oven.
14. Bake for about 15-17 minutes.
15. Remove the baking dish and sheet from the oven and let it cool for about 5 minutes before serving.

16. Top the casserole with the crispy onion slices evenly.
17. Cut into 6 equal-sized portions and serve.

Nutrition: calories 190, fat 2, carbs 18, protein 32

185. Vegetarian Pie

Preparation time: 20 minutes

Cooking Time: 1 hour 20 minutes

Servings: 8

Ingredients:

For Topping:

- 5 cups water
- 1¼ cups yellow cornmeal

For Filing:

- 1 tbsp extra-virgin olive oil
- 1 large onion, chopped
- 1 medium red bell pepper, seeded and chopped
- 2 garlic cloves, minced
- 1 tsp dried oregano, crushed
- 2 tsp chili powder
- 2 cups fresh tomatoes, chopped
- 2½ cups cooked pinto beans
- 2 cups boiled corn kernels

Directions:

1. Preheat the oven to 375 degrees F. Lightly grease a shallow baking dish.
2. In a pan, add the water over medium-high heat and bring to a boil.
3. Slowly, add the cornmeal, stirring continuously.
4. Reduce the heat to low and cook covered for about 20 minutes, stirring occasionally.
5. Meanwhile, prepare the filling. In a large skillet, heat the oil over medium heat and sauté the onion and bell pepper for about 3-4 minutes.
6. Add the garlic, oregano, and spices and sauté for about 1 minute

7. Add the remaining ingredients and stir to combine.
8. Reduce the heat to low and simmer for about 10-15 minutes, stirring occasionally.
9. Remove from the heat.
10. Place half of the cooked cornmeal into the prepared baking dish evenly.
11. Place the filling mixture over the cornmeal evenly.
12. Place the remaining cornmeal over the filling mixture evenly.
13. Bake for 45-50 minutes or until the top becomes golden brown.
14. Remove the pie from the oven and set it aside for about 5 minutes before serving.

Nutrition: calories 176, fat 1, carbs 10, protein 22

186. Rice & Lentil Loaf

Preparation time: 20 minutes

Cooking Time: 1 hour 50 minutes

Servings: 8

Ingredients:

- 1¾ cups plus 2 tbsp filtered water, divided
- ½ cup wild rice
- ½ cup brown lentils
- Pinch of sea salt
- ½ tsp no-sodium Italian seasoning
- 1 medium yellow onion, chopped
- 1 celery stalk, chopped
- 6 cremini mushrooms, chopped
- 4 garlic cloves, minced
- ¾ cup rolled oats
- ½ cup pecans, chopped finely
- ¾ cup homemade tomato sauce
- ½ tsp red pepper flakes, crushed
- 1 tsp fresh rosemary, minced
- 2 tsp fresh thyme, minced

Directions:

1. In a pan, add 1¾ cups of water, rice, lentils, salt, and Italian seasoning and bring them to a boil over medium-high heat.
2. Reduce the heat to low and simmer covered for about 45 minutes.
3. Remove from the heat and set it aside still covered for at least 10 minutes.
4. Preheat the oven to 350 degrees F.
5. With parchment paper, line a 9x5-inch loaf pan.
6. In a skillet, heat the remaining water over medium heat and sauté the onion, celery, mushrooms, and garlic for about 4-5 minutes.
7. Remove from the heat and let it cool slightly.
8. In a large mixing bowl, add the oats, pecans, tomato sauce, and fresh herbs and mix until well combined.
9. Combine the rice mixture and vegetable mixture with the oat mixture and mix well.
10. In a blender, add the mixture and pulse until a chunky mixture forms.
11. Transfer the mixture into the prepared loaf pan evenly.
12. With a piece of foil, cover the loaf pan and bake it for about 40 minutes.
13. Uncover and bake for about 15-20 minutes more or until the top becomes golden brown.
14. Remove it from the oven and set it aside for about 5-10 minutes before slicing.
15. Cut into desired sized slices and serve.

Nutrition: calories 220, fat 3, carbs 8, protein 21

187. Quinoa & Chickpea Salad

Preparation time: 15 minutes

Cooking time: 45 minutes

Servings: 8

Ingredients:

- 1¾ cups homemade vegetable broth
- 1 cup quinoa, rinsed
- Sea salt, to taste
- 1½ cups cooked chickpeas

- 1 medium green bell pepper, seeded and chopped
- 1 medium red bell pepper, seeded and chopped
- 2 cucumbers, chopped
- ½ cup scallion (green part only), chopped
- 1 tablespoon olive oil
- 2 tablespoons fresh cilantro leaves, chopped

Directions:

1. In a pan, add the broth and bring to a boil over high heat.
2. Add the quinoa and salt and cook until boiling again.
3. Reduce the heat to low and simmer covered for about 15-20 minutes or until all the liquid is absorbed.
4. Remove from the heat and set aside still covered for about 5-10 minutes.
5. Uncover and fluff the quinoa with a fork.
6. In a large serving bowl, add the quinoa and the remaining ingredients and gently toss to coat.
7. Serve immediately.

Nutrition: calories 276, fat 3, carbs 18, protein 28

188. Mixed Veggie Soup

Preparation time: 20 minutes

Cooking Time: 20 minutes.

Servings: 6

Ingredients:

- 1½ tablespoons olive oil
- 4 medium carrots, peeled and chopped
- 1 medium onion, chopped
- 2 garlic cloves, minced
- 2 celery stalks, chopped
- 2 cups fresh tomatoes, chopped finely
- 3 cups small cauliflower florets
- 3 cups small broccoli florets
- 3 cups frozen peas

- 8 cups homemade vegetable broth
- 3 tablespoons fresh lemon juice
- Sea salt, to taste

Directions:

1. In a large soup pan, heat the oil over medium heat and sauté the carrots, celery, and onion for 6 minutes.
2. Stir in the garlic and sauté for about 1 minute.
3. Add the tomatoes and cook for about 2-3 minutes, crushing them with the back of a spoon.
4. Add the vegetables and broth and bring to a boil over high heat.
5. Reduce the heat to low.
6. Cover the pan and simmer for about 30-35 minutes.
7. Mix in the lemon juice and salt and remove from the heat.
8. Serve hot.

Nutrition: calories 173, fat 5, carbs 18, protein 19

189. Beans & Barley Soup

Preparation time: 15 minutes

Cooking time: 40 minutes

Servings: 4

Ingredients:

- 1 tablespoon olive oil
- 1 white onion, chopped
- 2 celery stalks, chopped
- 1 large carrot, peeled and chopped
- 2 tablespoons fresh rosemary, chopped
- 2 garlic cloves, minced
- 4 cups fresh tomatoes, chopped
- 4 cups homemade vegetable broth
- 1 cup pearl barley
- 2 cups cooked white beans
- 2 tablespoons fresh lemon juice

- 4 tablespoons fresh parsley leaves, chopped

Directions:

1. In a large soup pan, heat the oil over medium heat and sauté the onion, celery, and carrot for about 4-5 minutes.
2. Add the garlic and rosemary and sauté for about 1 minute.
3. Add the tomatoes and cook for 3-4 minutes, crushing them with the back of a spoon.
4. Add the barley and broth and bring to a boil.
5. Reduce the heat to low and simmer covered for about 20-25 minutes.
6. Stir in the beans and lemon juice and simmer for about 5 minutes more.
7. Garnish with parsley and serve hot

Nutrition: calories 278, fat 13, carbs 8, protein 19

190. Tofu & Bell Pepper Stew

Preparation time: 15 minutes

Cooking time: 15 minutes

Servings: 6

Ingredients:

- 2 tablespoons garlic
- 1 jalapeño pepper, seeded and chopped
- 1 (16-ounce) jar roasted red peppers, rinsed, drained, and chopped
- 2 cups homemade vegetable broth
- 2 cups filtered water
- 1 medium green bell pepper, seeded and sliced thinly
- 1 medium red bell pepper, seeded and sliced thinly
- 1 (16-ounce) package extra-firm tofu, drained and cubed
- 1 (10-ounce) package frozen baby spinach, thawed

Directions:

1. Add the garlic, jalapeño pepper, and roasted red peppers in a food processor and pulse until smooth.

2. In a large pan, add the puree, broth, and water and cook until boiling over medium-high heat.
3. Add the bell peppers and tofu and stir to combine.
4. Reduce the heat to medium and cook for about 5 minutes.
5. Stir in the spinach and cook for about 5 minutes.
6. Serve hot.

Nutrition: calories 111, fat 7, carbs 9, protein 18

191. Lentils with Kale

Preparation time: 15 minutes

Cooking time: 20 minutes

Servings: 6

Ingredients:

- 1½ cups red lentils
- 1½ cups homemade vegetable broth
- 1½ tablespoons olive oil
- ½ cup onion, chopped
- 1 teaspoon fresh ginger, peeled and minced
- 2 garlic cloves, minced
- 1½ cups tomato, chopped
- 6 cups fresh kale, tough ends removed and chopped
- Sea salt and ground black pepper, to taste

Directions:

1. In a pan, add the broth and lentils and bring to a boil over medium-high heat.
2. Reduce the heat to low and simmer covered for about 20 minutes or until almost all the liquid is absorbed.
3. Remove from the heat and set aside still covered.
4. Meanwhile, in a large skillet, heat oil over medium heat and sauté the onion for about 5-6 minutes.
5. Add the ginger and garlic and sauté for about 1 minute.
6. Add tomatoes and kale and cook for about 4-5 minutes.

7. Stir in the lentils, salt, and black pepper then remove from heat.
8. Serve hot.

Nutrition: calories 188, fat 4, carbs 6, protein 11

192. Veggie Ratatouille

Preparation time: 20 minutes

Cooking time: 45 minutes 5 minutes

Servings: 4

Ingredients:

- 6 ounces homemade tomato paste
- 3 tablespoons olive oil, divided
- ½ of an onion, chopped
- 3 tablespoons garlic, minced
- Sea salt and freshly ground black pepper, to taste
- ¾ cup filtered water
- 1 eggplant, sliced into thin circles
- 1 red bell pepper, seeded and sliced into thin circles
- 1 yellow bell pepper, seeded and sliced into thin circles
- 1 tablespoon fresh thyme leaves, minced
- 1 tablespoon fresh lemon juice

Directions:

1. Preheat oven to 375 degrees F.
2. In a bowl, add the tomato paste, 1 tablespoon of oil, onion, garlic, salt, and black pepper and mix nicely.
3. In the bottom of a 10x10-inch baking dish, spread the tomato paste mixture evenly.
4. Arrange alternating vegetable slices starting at the outer edge of the baking dish and working concentrically towards the center.
5. Drizzle the remaining oil and lemon juice over the vegetables and sprinkle them with salt and black pepper followed by the thyme.
6. Arrange a piece of parchment paper over the vegetables.
7. Bake for about 45 minutes.

8. Serve hot.

Nutrition: calories 143, fat 4, carbs 7, protein 19

193. Baked Beans

Preparation time: 15 minutes

Cooking time: 2 hours 5 minutes

Servings: 4

Ingredients:

- ¼ pound dry lima beans, soaked overnight and drained
- ¼ pound dry red kidney beans, soaked overnight and drained
- 1¼ tablespoons olive oil
- 1 small yellow onion, chopped
- 4 garlic cloves, minced
- 1 teaspoon dried thyme, crushed
- ½ teaspoon ground cumin
- ½ teaspoon red pepper flakes, crushed
- ¼ teaspoon smoked paprika
- 1 tablespoon fresh lemon juice
- 1 cup homemade tomato sauce
- 1 cup homemade vegetable broth

Directions:

1. Add the beans to a large pan of boiling water and bring back to a boil.
2. Reduce the heat to low.
3. Cover the pan and cook for about 1 hour.
4. Drain the beans well.
5. Preheat the oven to 325 degrees F.
6. In a large oven-proof pan, heat the oil over medium heat and sauté the onion for about 4 minutes.
7. Add the garlic, thyme, and spices, and sauté for about 1 minute.
8. Stir in the cooked beans and remaining ingredients and immediately remove from the heat.
9. Cover the pan and bake in oven for about 1 hour.

10. Serve hot.

Nutrition: calories 160, fat 2, carbs 7, protein 19

194. Cannellini Bean Cashew Dip

Preparation time: 1 hour

Cooking time: 1 hour

Servings: 8

Ingredients:

- 1 15-ounce can cannellini beans, rinsed and drained
- ½ cup raw cashews
- 1 clove garlic, smashed
- 2 tablespoons diced, red bell pepper
- ½ teaspoon sea salt
- ¼ teaspoon cayenne pepper
- 4 teaspoons lemon juice
- 2 tablespoons water
- Dill sprigs or weed for garnish

Directions:

1. Place the beans, cashews, garlic, and bell pepper in the food processor and pulse several times to break it up.
2. Add the salt, cayenne, lemon juice, and water and process until smooth.
3. Scrape into a bowl, cover, and refrigerate for at least an hour before serving.
4. Garnish with fresh dill and serve with vegetables, crackers, or pita chips.

Nutrition: calories 132, fat 6, carbs 9, protein 18

195. Cauliflower Popcorn

Preparation time: 1 day and 1 hour

Cooking time: 1 day

Servings: 2

Ingredients:

- ¼ cup sun-dried tomatoes
- ¾ cup dates
- 2 heads cauliflower
- ½ cup water
- 2 tablespoons raw tahini
- 1 tablespoon apple cider vinegar
- 2 teaspoons onion powder
- 2 teaspoons garlic powder
- 1 teaspoon ground cayenne pepper
- 2 tablespoons nutritional yeast (optional)

Directions:

1. Cover the sun-dried tomatoes with warm water and let them soak for an hour.
2. If the dates are not soft and fresh, soak them in warm water for an hour in another bowl.
3. Cut the cauliflower into very small, bite-sized pieces then set aside.
4. Put the drained tomatoes and dates in a blender along with the water, tahini, apple cider vinegar, onion powder, garlic powder, cayenne pepper, nutritional yeast, and turmeric. Blend into a thick, smooth consistency.
5. Pour this mixture into the bowl, atop the cauliflower, and mix so that all the pieces are coated.
6. Place the cauliflower in the dehydrator and spread it out to make a single layer. Sprinkle with a little sea salt and set for 115 degrees, Fahrenheit for 12 to 24 hours or until it becomes exactly as crunchy as you like it. I let mine go for 15 to 16 hours, but the time will vary based on your taste preference as well as the ambient humidity.
7. Store in an airtight container until serving.

Nutrition: calories 170, fat 2, carbs 6, protein 16

196. Cinnamon Apple Chips with Dip

Preparation time: 3 hours and 30 minutes

Cooking time: 3 hours

Servings: 2

Ingredients:

- 1 cup raw cashews
- 2 apples, thinly sliced
- 1 lemon
- 1½ cups water, divided
- Cinnamon plus more to dust the chips
- Another medium cored apple quartered
- 1 tablespoon honey or agave
- 1 teaspoon cinnamon
- ¼ teaspoon sea salt

Directions:

1. Place the cashews in a bowl of warm water, deep enough to cover them, and let them soak overnight.
2. Preheat the oven to 200 degrees, Fahrenheit. Line two baking sheets with parchment paper.
3. Juice the lemon into a large glass bowl and add two cups of the water. Place the sliced apples in the water as you cut them and when done, swish them around and drain.
4. Spread the apple slices across the baking sheet in a single layer and sprinkle with a little cinnamon. Bake for 90 minutes.
5. Remove the slices from the oven and flip each of them over. Put them back in the oven and bake for another 90 minutes, or until they are crisp. Remember, they will get crisper as they cool.
6. While the apple slices are cooking, drain the cashews and put them in a blender, along with the quartered apple, the honey, a teaspoon of cinnamon, and a half cup of the remaining water. Process until thick and creamy. I like

to refrigerate my dip for about an hour to chill before serving alongside the room temperature apple slices.

Nutrition: calories 190, fat 1, carbs 18, protein 32

197. Crunchy Asparagus Spears

Preparation time: 25 minutes

Cooking time: 25 minutes

Servings: 4

Ingredients:

- 1 bunch asparagus spears (about 12 spears)
- ¼ cup nutritional yeast
- 2 tablespoons hemp seeds
- 1 teaspoon garlic powder
- ¼ teaspoon paprika (or more if you like paprika)
- ⅛ teaspoon ground pepper
- ¼ cup whole-wheat breadcrumbs
- Juice of ½ lemon

Directions:

1. Preheat the oven to 350 degrees, Fahrenheit. Line a baking sheet with parchment paper.
2. Wash the asparagus, snapping off the white part at the bottom. Save it for making vegetable stock.
3. Mix together the nutritional yeast, hemp seed, garlic powder, paprika, pepper, and breadcrumbs.
4. Place asparagus spears on the baking sheets giving them a little room in between and sprinkle with the mixture in the bowl.
5. Bake for up to 25 minutes, until crispy.
6. Serve with lemon juice if desired.

Nutrition: calories 156, fat 4, carbs 7, protein 18

198. Cucumber Bites with Chive and Sunflower Seeds

Preparation time: 5 minutes

Cooking time: 5 minutes

Servings: 2

Ingredients:

- 1 cup raw sunflower seed
- ½ teaspoon salt
- ½ cup chopped fresh chives
- 1 clove garlic, chopped
- 2 tablespoons red onion, minced
- 2 tablespoons lemon juice
- ½ cup water (might need more or less)
- 4 large cucumbers

Directions:

1. Place the sunflower seeds and salt in the food processor and process to a fine powder. It will take only about 10 seconds.
2. Add the chives, garlic, onion, lemon juice, and water and process until creamy, scraping down the sides frequently. The mixture should be very creamy; if not, add a little more water.
3. Cut the cucumbers into 1½-inch coin-like pieces.
4. Spread a spoonful of the sunflower mixture on top and set on a platter. Sprinkle more chopped chives on top and refrigerate until ready to serve.

Nutrition: calories 177, fat 1, carbs 8, protein 16

199. Garlicky Kale Chips

Preparation time: 1 hour and 30 min

Cooking time: 1 hour

Servings: 2

Ingredients:

- 4 cloves garlic
- 1 cup olive oil
- 8 to 10 cups fresh kale, chopped
- 1 tablespoon of garlic-flavored olive oil
- ½ teaspoon garlic salt
- ½ teaspoon pepper
- 1 pinch red pepper flakes (optional)

Directions:

1. Peel and crush the garlic clove and place it in a small jar with a lid. Pour the olive oil over the top, cover tightly, and shake. This will keep in the refrigerator for several days. When you're ready to use it, strain out the garlic and retain the oil.
2. Preheat the oven to 175 degrees, Fahrenheit.
3. Spread out the kale on a baking sheet and drizzle with the olive oil. Sprinkle with garlic salt, pepper, and red pepper flakes.
4. Bake for an hour, remove from the oven, and let the chips cool.
5. Store in an airtight container if you don't plan to eat them right away.

Nutrition: calories 211, fat 3, carbs 18, protein 21

200. Hummus-Stuffed Baby Potatoes

Preparation time: 30 minutes

Cooking time: 30 minutes

Servings: 2

Ingredients:

- 12 small red potatoes, walnut-sized or slightly larger
- Hummus
- 2 green onions, thinly sliced
- ¼ teaspoon paprika, for garnish

Directions:

1. Place two to three inches of water in a saucepan, set a steamer inside, and bring the water to a boil.
2. Place the whole potatoes in the steamer basket and steam for about 20 minutes or until soft. Keep the pan from boiling dry by adding additional hot water as needed.
3. Dump the potatoes into a colander and run cold water over them until they can be handled.
4. Cut each potato open and scoop out most of the pulp, leaving the skin and a thin layer of potato intact.
5. Mix the hummus with most of the green onions (keep enough for garnish) and spoon a little into the area where the potato has been scooped out.
6. Sprinkle each filled potato half with paprika and serve.

Nutrition: calories 329, fat 3, carbs 8, protein 14

Chapter 14

HOW MUCH YOU MUST DRINK AND WHY IT IS SO IMPORTANT

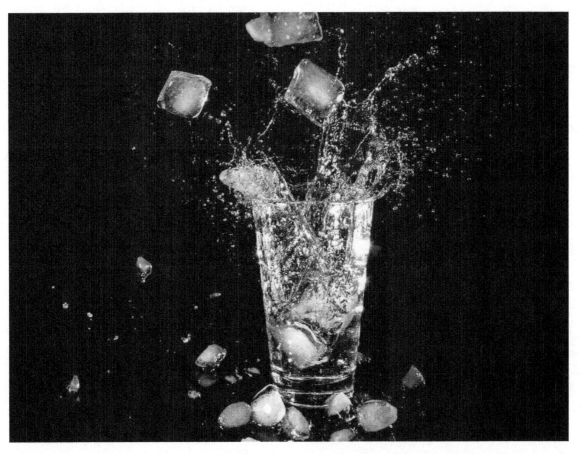

Enough liquid in the body, especially warm liquid, can help drain the sinuses and thin the mucus. Thus, drinking large amounts of water can help clear out mucus from the body. Dr. Sebi recommends a high intake of water. Also, most fruits and vegetables recommended by Dr. Sebi's diet have high water content. These foods help to keep the body hydrated and prevent excess mucus production.

Moreover, some drinks like coffee and alcohol can cause dehydration in the body. Anyone on the Dr. Sebi diet must stay away from alcohol. This helps to avoid dehydration.

Action: Take a lot of water, smoothies, and juice made with Dr. Sebi's approved foods.

Expectorants

Expectorants are known to help in clearing mucus. Expectorants loosen and thin mucus, which makes it easy to cough it out of the system. There are some herbs in the Dr. Sebi diet which can serve as expectorants. The most used herb of Dr. Sebi's approved herbs is the Red Clover.

Red Clover is a super healthy herb which aids circulation in the body. It is a natural blood purifier, and also serves as an expectorant. It is widely used by women in treating menopause-related conditions like hot flashes and lumbar spine protection. So, taking red clover can help to loosen and clear mucus from the body.

Action: In 8 oz of hot water, steep 1 - 2 teaspoons of the dried flower and allow for up to 30 minutes. Then drink at least 2 and not more than 3 cups per day. Or, sip 1ml of the fluid extract with hot water three times daily.

Essential Oils

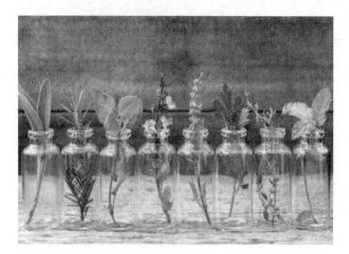

Some essential oils have been proposed to be very effective in the treatment of lung disease-related symptoms. People use essential oils for the treatment and prevention of chest cold and sinusitis. Some of these essential oils can be gotten from Dr. Sebi approved products like eucalyptus, oregano, and thyme.

Eucalyptus has been widely used for many years to treat coughs and reduce mucus production. It helps to loosen the mucus so it can be easily coughed out. Thus, it relieves nagging coughs.

Action: Make your own homemade vapor rub by adding 12 drops of eucalyptus oil to ¼ cup of coconut oil. Alternatively, add 1 drop of eucalyptus oil to 1 teaspoon of water.

First test the mixture to know whether it is safe for use. Then apply it directly on your skin, especially on your throat and chest. This makes the scents easily reach the nose and mouth.

CONCLUSION

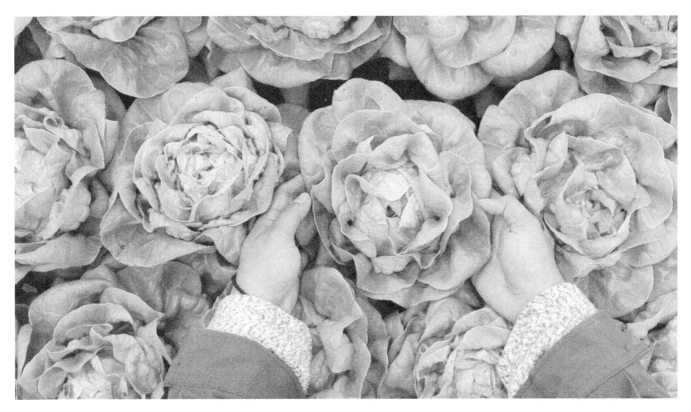

Thank you for making it to the end of the **Dr. Sebi Diet Recipes** book. 'Health is wealth,' many will say, but still, they neglect the call to give proper attention to their health for numerous reasons. Top of the list mostly is the lack of time, but when we are struck by sickness, time eventually pauses because we cannot do what we want. We fail to understand that illnesses and diseases accumulate over time, they do not just appear from nowhere. Your body must have been giving you signs, but you ignored them all.

When you start feeling tired easily, experiencing digestive distress, your allergies become more frequent, you start feeling unhealthy despite eating well, feel weak in your joints, not mentally sharp as usual, and you feel stressed out easily, etc., that is your body sending you a message. This can be likened to a car before it breaks down. It always gives off signals, like starting after several attempts, jerking, and making some weird sounds. These signals are your defense mechanism reacting to the anomalies or impending danger posed by pathogens. So, when we get these signals, we ought to act almost immediately to ensure that our body system gets back to normal.

Most times, the simple thing to do is detox, which is to rid our system of unwanted materials.

Printed in Great Britain
by Amazon